The Chiropractic Way To Health

"The Ultimate Self-Help Guide For Chiropractic Patients"

The
Chiropractic
Way To Health

"The Ultimate Self-Help Guide For Chiropractic Patients"

Dr. Anita Haque

Indialantic Publishing

Published by Indialantic Publishing, 1291-M Folly Road, Charleston, South Carolina 29412. Member of the Indialantic Publishing Group.

Printed in the United States of America

Design by Paul Dolphin

Photographs by Matthew Scott: pgs: 59 (bottom photo), 64, 65 (bottom photo), 67, 68, 70, 130 (bottom photo), 134 (bottom photo), 138, 139 (top photo), 140, 141, 152 (bottom photo), 157, 158

Photographs by Tom Anastasion: pgs: 42, 43, 44, 45, 46, 49, 54, 55, 56, 57 (top two photos), 65 (top two photos), 66, 71, 121

Photographs by Don Taylor: pgs: 111, 112, 113, 114, 115, 116, 117, 118, 129, 130 (top photo), 131, 132, 133, 134 (top photo), 135, 136, 137, 142, 143, 144, 145, 146, 147, 148, 149, 150, 151, 153, 160, 169, 170 171, 172, 173, 174

Grateful acknowledgment is made to the following for permission to reprint illustrations and photographs: Paul Dolphin for the original illustrations on pages 18, 101 and 151 (top), Palmer College of Chiropractic Archives, David D. Palmer Health Sciences Library: pgs. 2 (both photos) and 19, Istock: pg. 175.

Disclaimer

The exercises and advice contained within this book may be too strenuous or dangerous for some people, and the reader(s) should consult a physician before engaging in them.

The author and publisher of this book are not responsible in any manner whatsoever for any injury which may occur through reading and following the instructions herein.

To Don Parker, Anjum and Anwar Haque and Reena Shah.
You are the lights of my life.

CONTENTS

Acknowledgments

Thank you to all of my chiropractic colleagues past and present, here in the United States and around the world, who are working to develop and spread the greatest healing art in the world.

Special thanks to the following chiropractors, who've shared their knowledge and enthusiasm with me: Dr. Chuck Gibson, Dr. Stacey Gillis, Dr. Marianne Abate, Dr. Scott Beavers, Dr. Sheena Sohl and Dr. Erich Breitenmoser.

I'm also grateful to my staff at Haque Chiropractic, Inc.in Livermore, CA including Don Parker, Sandy Kleinpeter, and all other members of Lifestyle Fitness and Haque Chiropractic, Inc.

It's with great love and appreciation that I extend the warmest thanks to all of my patients, without whom this book would not have been possible.

The Chiropractic Way To Health

"The Ultimate Self-Help Guide For Chiropractic Patients"

INTRODUCTION

Most people think chiropractors deal with relieving back pain, neck pain and headaches. The truth is, chiropractic started by helping people with much more serious problems.

It was September 18, 1895 in Davenport, Iowa. Harvey Lillard, who was deaf, was working as a janitor, cleaning the offices of Dr. D.D. Palmer. Palmer knew that Lillard had not always been deaf, because the man could speak. The doctor inquired how he had lost his hearing (perhaps he wrote on a slip of paper, perhaps Lillard could read his lips).

Lillard said he had been working in a stooped position one day when something "gave" in his back. Soon afterwards, his hearing faded. Palmer asked Lillard if he might examine him and the janitor agreed, lying down. A large lump could be seen on his neck. It appeared as though a bone there had become misaligned.

Palmer received permission to try putting the bone back into place. Placing his hands on Lillard's spine, the doctor gave a thrust. There was a soft pop.

It was a hot day in Davenport and the windows were open. Lillard got off the table. His eyes grew wide as he went to the windows and leaned out. "Dr. Palmer!" he cried. "I can hear the wagon wheels on the cobblestone!" With one spinal adjustment, Lillard recovered his hearing.

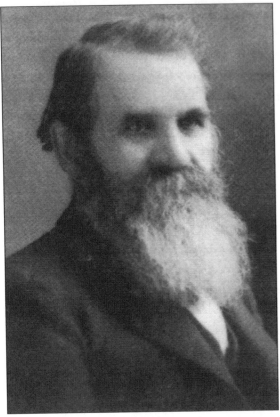

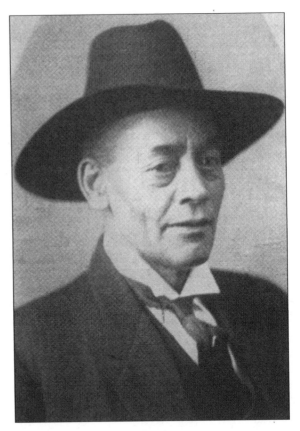

D.D Palmer

Harvey Lillard

Palmer first thought he had discovered a cure for deafness but soon realized something else was at work.

"Shortly after this relief from deafness, I had a case of heart trouble which was not improving," Palmer later wrote. "I examined the spine and found a displaced vertebra pressing against the nerves which innervate (go to) the heart. I adjusted the vertebra and gave immediate relief. Then I began to reason that if two diseases, so dissimilar as deafness and heart trouble, came from impingement, a pressure on nerves, were not other diseases due to a similar cause?"

Palmer began developing his "hand treatments," and was soon getting results with many different conditions—asthma, colic, ear infections, digestion problems, neck and back pains, headaches—virtually any ailment might be a candidate for the new healing art. Soon people from all over the country were traveling to Davenport for spinal adjustments.

Reverend Samuel Weed, one of Palmer's first patients, gave the new profession a name. He took the Greek word for "hand' (cheir) and "done by" (praktos), combining them into "chiropractic," meaning, "done by hand".

D.D. went on to found the Palmer School of Chiropractic in Davenport, and the profession grew quickly. Today there are more than 60,000 chiropractors across the globe.

Chiropractic is a philosophy, art and science of things natural...a system by which the flow of life is released and increased in your body...a plan of living, involving in its makeup everything that is essential to the vigorous and healthful performance of all the functions of life.

More than two dozen colleges worldwide graduate thousands of spinal experts each year, making chiropractic the fastest growing health care profession in the world. According to Time magazine, one out of 20 people will visit a chiropractor this year, and this number is expected to double in the next ten years.

Chiropractic is growing so fast because it works. People are also realizing that drugs and surgery, while necessary at times, aren't the best ways to get or stay healthy. As one of my friends says, "If drugs are so dangerous to take when you're pregnant, why do doctors want to give them to our children?" Another likes to ask his patients considering surgery, "Have you ever cut anything that made it more whole?"

Ask yourself, "Do I want more drugs and surgeries in my life?" Most people answer no, realizing medical intervention only attempts to fix ill health. I often pose this question to patients: "Can you imagine walking into your local emergency room and saying, "Listen, I feel fantastic today and I want to feel better. Check me in!"

Medicine's focus on treating problems keeps it from being a tool we can use to attain total wellness and peak performance. In my clinic, if a "healthy" person comes in and wants to get healthier, I can virtually guarantee them that under chiropractic care they will experience more energy, better digestion, better sleep, increased athletic performance and fewer colds and diseases.

A chiropractor shared this story with me recently: His mother-in-law died after a six-week stay in a major hospital's intensive care unit. Several "heroic" surgeries were attempted to save the woman's life, to no avail. Her bill for six weeks in the hospital: $400,000.

The chiropractor said, "What if my mother-in-law were able to take $400,000 when she was 21-years-old and invested it in her health? What if she joined the best health club, ate the most wholesome foods and enjoyed chiropractic care to keep her body in top shape? Do you realize it would be nearly impossible to spend $400,000 in your lifetime on staying healthy, yet you can spend it in six weeks on being sick!"

One of our biggest problems in health care is that we're spending huge amounts treating sickness and disease instead of promoting health within ourselves. There's a saying, "It's better to help the good than fight the bad." Chiropractic can help our bodies work better.

Millions have already discovered this. Today every professional football, basketball, baseball and hockey team is associated with a chiropractor, whose job is to help million-dollar players perform at their peak.

Joe Montana, the former star quarterback who many think is the best that's ever played the game, credits chiropractic with helping him play his best.

"The way I look at it is that it makes me feel better, I'm healthier, and it keeps me on the field," said Montana several years before retiring. "Chiropractic isn't just for a bad back or neck. It's about prevention so your body can function at optimum health. I don't see any reason why I shouldn't do it." Montana's entire family receives regular chiropractic spinal adjustments. Other top athletes like Tiger Woods in golf and Lance Armstrong in cycling get adjusted before, after and sometimes during competitions.

Celebrities such as Mel Gibson, Bruce Willis, Madonna, Demi Moore, Racquel Welch and Arnold Schwarzenegger are all enthusiastic chiropractic patients. But you don't have to be a movie star or professional athlete to benefit from chiropractic. It's for you, too. In the chapters ahead you'll find advice based on chiropractic's principle of helping your body function at 100 percent by eliminating what D. D. Palmer termed "pressure on nerves".

What about drugs?

Bernard Detmar, M.D., Ph.D., had this to say about drugs:

The use of drugs is an emergency aid. Drugs never heal. Only the patient's constitution can do that. Regular use of drugs, not to speak of excessive use, so weakens the body's powers of resistance that it finally succumbs. Generally speaking the weaker the dose of a drug, the less harm it causes."

All drugs are designed to treat symptoms, not to correct causes. There is no drug without harmful side effects. And the more powerful the drug the more powerful the side effects.

Another consideration: Drug interactions. If you mix two known chemicals in a beaker in a laboratory the results are predictable. *Your* body chemistry, however, is unique and constantly changing. So when you add one, two, five or ten drugs to this unknown environment there is NO WAY to know what will happen.

This is why adverse drug reactions are among the top ten causes of death in the United States each year. The fewer drugs you take, the better.

Natural Healthcare. . .

"Chiropractic is about natural, preventive health care. There's nothing that fits better together than chiropractic and weight training and sports and fitness, because it all has to do with this: how do we make our bodies healthier, how do we become more energetic, more powerful, more flexible and how to create longevity? I have experienced this for the last 20 years myself on my own body. Whenever I have a problem—or even if I don't have a problem—I go to my chiropractor. Dr. Franco Columbu is a great chiropractor and he has been with me for so many years, in competitions, in making movies; he is like my own personal chiropractor, always there to take care of me, and that has been a big part of my success."

--Arnold Schwarzenegger

5

Benefits of Chiropractic Care

**Following are just some of the benefits of chiropractic care
reported by millions of chiropractic patients:**

Relief from:

- Ankle/foot pain
- Carpel tunnel syndrome and hand/wrist pain
- Degenerative joint disease in the neck and low back
- Dizziness/vertigo
- Elbow pain
- Headaches, both common and migraine
- Herniated or "slipped" discs
- Hip, knee and ankle problems
- Jaw (TMJ) problems
- Knee pain
- Low back pain
- Neck pain, including the pain from whiplash-type injuries suffered in auto accidents
- Menstrual pain
- Sciatica (pain down the leg)
- Shoulder problems
- Many other common—and not so common—health problems

Improvements in:

- Blood supply to the brain, making for better concentration and reduced feelings of anxiety, depression and fatigue
- Circulation
- Diabetic conditions
- Energy levels
- Digestion
- Immune system function
- Lung/breathing functions
- Sleep

1 A NEW VIEW OF HEALTH

[health is an inside job]

Talking Health

Most people think health is "feeling good". In other words, if they wake up in the morning without pain or other symptoms, they're healthy. It turns out, surprisingly to many people, that this is not the best way to measure your health.

A Clean Bill of Health

Ironically, the reason most people get less and less healthy as the years go by is that they believe this: "If I feel good, I must be healthy." This reasoning is why most middle-aged men and women carry aches and pains in their bodies the way suitcases carry clothing. It's why many senior citizens spend their last years battling degenerative diseases like arthritis, high blood pressure and heart disease, and why so many die untimely deaths.

Feeling good doesn't mean you're healthy. For example, according to "Boyd's Pathology," a standard textbook in virtually all medical schools, in most cases it takes years before cancer cells in the breast grow to a lump you can feel during self-examination. This means a woman could be doing self-exams for years, finding nothing, while in fact cancer is growing beneath her fingertips. She might feel great. But is she healthy?

Cancer often takes its victims by surprise, but what about something as common--and deadly--as a heart attack? Surely almost everyone with heart problems has early indications there is trouble brewing. Nope. In many cases the first "symptom" of a heart attack is death. In other words, many times the person just drops dead. We've all heard stories of "healthy" middle-aged men doing a common chore like mowing the lawn when they suffer a massive heart attack.

Such commonplace stories shock us. They slap us in the face with a simple fact: A pain-free body isn't necessarily healthy. They also reveal a basic truth: **While feeling good is often a benefit of health, it's not what health is.**

So where did we get this idea that health is merely "feeling good"? The answer is as close as your medicine cabinet.

Can't Buy Me Health

The United States is rich with more medical doctors than any other country in the world. We have more hospitals, too. And more than half of the medical "breakthroughs" in treating disease take place right here.

We're spending vast amounts of money on health care. What does it buy? One thing: *quality emergency health care.* If you're shot, if your parachute doesn't open, or if you're otherwise burnt, broken or torn, there's no better place to be treated than in the United States. Modern medicine also is good at things like kidney transplants and hip replacements—cutting out or replacing body parts that have lost their ability to function.

Is there anything our expensive medical establishment **doesn't** buy? The World Health Organization (WHO) ranks countries for overall health. Where do we rank? In the early 1930s the U.S. ranked second in overall health. Sadly, since then we've been dropping faster than a spoon through hot soup. Today over 30 countries rank higher in overall health even though more of our Gross Domestic Product goes toward health care than any other country in the world. For all the money we spend, people in many other countries enjoy a longer life span.

How can we be swamped with doctors, hospitals and high-tech medicine and yet be getting less and less healthy?

Recent statistics show that, on average, all Americans, even those with good health insurance, are getting less healthy. It's now estimated that one in four will develop heart disease. One in five will die of cancer. The most appalling fact is that young people today are less healthy than at any time since the turn of the century.

When I discuss these facts with patients they will explain our predicament in a number of ways. Many say, "It's our lifestyle."

"We eat too much."

"We don't exercise enough."

"We're under too much stress."

These are all valid explanations. But there's something more basic. Why do so many live in a way that creates aching bodies filled with disease?

The Misinformation Age

We live in a time when there's never been more information in books, magazines, newspapers, the Internet, etc. about how to get healthy (get regular exercise, eat low fat, low salt food, don't smoke, etc.) But most people still--lack a basic understanding of what, exactly, is this thing called health. Why?

The Drug Connection

According to CBS' *"60 Minutes,"* pharmaceutical companies spend more than $1 billion per month on advertising and promotion. That's more than is spent researching and developing their products. About one fifth of all television commercials advertise drugs. By the time the average child reaches 18, he or she has seen *20,000* hours of drug commercials.

All that marketing pays off. Americans now take more than half of all the drugs in the world, swallowing or injecting about 25 million doses each hour. There are more than 25,000 prescription potions and 200,000 over-the-counter drugs on the market, with the average American home containing 29 different types.

My favorite drug commercial targets, as it says, "the person who needs a pain reliever several times a week." It begins by showing a pretty, smartly dressed young woman in her kitchen, cooking breakfast. The bottom of the television screen reads, "Monday Morning". It's the kind of day we'd all like to enjoy at the start of a week. Sunlight is pouring through a large picture window. You can almost hear the birds outside, chirping merrily. Suddenly, the woman's son comes running through the kitchen. In his enthusiasm he knocks over a pitcher of orange juice. In slow motion it falls, smashing on the floor. With glass flying everywhere the woman is seized by a terrible headache. She grabs her head. The camera zooms in. Her head pulsates. Ba-boom! Ba-boom! Ba-boom!, goes the soundtrack. Then she takes a pain reliever, and, ahhh...the pain goes away.

The commercial continues, but now the bottom of the screen reads "Wednesday Afternoon." The woman is bending over, picking grocery bags out of her car trunk. Wham! Suddenly she's seized by a terrible backache. She grabs her flank. It pulsates. The camera zooms in. Ba-boom! Ba-boom! Ba-boom! Again she takes a pain reliever, and the pain goes away.

This commercial's theme is repeated hundreds of times each day by other medicine makers. The message is always the same: As long as you can relieve the headache, backache, upset stomach, or vaginal yeast infection by taking a pill, syrup or caplet, or by applying a cream, gel or lotion, you're healthy again. In other words, *if you develop symptoms that make you feel bad, you're unhealthy. The way to get healthy again is to get rid of the symptoms.*

The Feeling Trap

We're brought up to believe that maintaining health is a matter of eliminating pesky symptoms. But **symptoms aren't the problem**. Symptoms only point to an underlying problem. Unless the true cause is corrected, symptoms come back or show up later in another, often more harmful, form.

If "the person who needs a pain reliever several times a week" would stop and think, they might say, "If I need to keep taking these pills all the time, are they really fixing anything?" The packages for pain relievers say, "For the temporary relief of pain." The reason they say *temporary* is because medications only mask pain while circulating in your blood. Once drugs get flushed from your body, the stage is set for more pain.

Put out the Fire or Knock the Alarm off the Wall?

If we treated our cars the same way we do our heads when we take aspirin for a headache, it might go something like this: You're on vacation, driving your car to another state. Suddenly your temperature gauge starts blinking red. The light is a symptom brought on by an overheated engine. Applying the same logic to your car as your head, you might take an aspirin bottle out of your pocket and cover the flashing light! You've taken care of the symptom, but have you solved the problem?

Do you know someone who takes a pain reliever every day for a headache or a backache? What if, tonight, you were awakened from a sound sleep by a fire alarm. You ran into the next room and there was a fire burning in the middle of the room. *Would you put out the fire or knock the alarm off the wall?* If you're taking a pain reliever every day for a headache or backache, you're knocking the alarm off the wall. Your body is trying to tell you something is wrong, and you're just quieting that symptom.

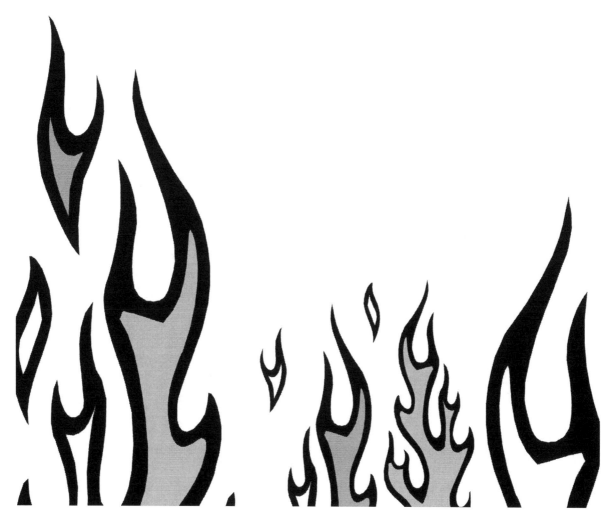

When Sick Is Healthy

Is there a healthier way to look at symptoms? Let's look at some typical symptoms associated with colds and flues. A list might look like this:

- Sneezing and coughing
- Diarrhea and vomiting
- Fatigue
- Loss of appetite
- Pain
- Fever

Why does your body sneeze and cough? Everyone knows it's to get rid of germs. In fact, with each cough or sneeze someone with the flu gets rid of thousands of germs from their body. Coughing also brings up mucus, produced as the body fights infection.

Is it good or bad that your body expels the germs infecting it? I think you'd agree it's good.

If you go to a Chinese restaurant and order Chow Mien, and along with it get Ptomaine poisoning, is it good or bad that your body quickly dumps the poison through vomiting and diarrhea? What would happen if you ate the poison and *couldn't* get rid of it?

If you're fighting an infection, should you spend the day in aerobics classes or eating a five-course lunch? Do you think you'd get better faster if you rested and let the energy usually used to digest food be put to use fighting your infection?

How about pain? Say you're hammering nails while listening to the radio. A song takes you back to a pleasant memory. Your mind drifts and...pow! You miss the nail and hit your thumb. A terrible pain shoots up your arm. Good or bad? What would happen if your thumb couldn't produce pain and you kept daydreaming? Pain lets us know something is wrong.

The body has a reason for creating fevers, too, which act to speed up the action of our immune systems: A university study traced two groups of children with measles. Half were untreated for fever, half given a medication to reduce their fevers. The group whose fevers were left to do their jobs recovered sooner.

Most people think that when they're sick and develop symptoms they're unhealthy. But when you're sick your body is actually working very hard through sneezing, coughing, diarrhea, vomiting, pain, fatigue and fever to get you well. All these symptoms are the body's' own ability to heal itself or a warning that something is wrong.

You would never guess your body has the ability to heal itself by watching drug commercials and observing our current medical system.

Chiropractors, on the other hand, recognize your body's ability to heal. Instead of treating symptoms, they remove the interference that prevents your healing powers from getting and keeping you well. When they do your body has a chance to recuperate.

When I talk with people about these ideas many say, "Oh, you're just against drugs because you're a chiropractor." It's not that I'm against all drugs all the time. What I'm concerned about is the idea that covering up or getting rid of symptoms allows us to gain full health, especially when talking about serious health problems.

For example, how about the person who is 70 pounds overweight, works at a high-stress job, doesn't exercise and eats enough fat each day to grease a roller coaster? After a decade or two of living this lifestyle they (surprise!) develop symptoms of high blood pressure. Many high-blood-pressure patients can cure themselves by eating a more nutritious diet, exercising regularly and learning to relax, which together take about a half hour per day. Or they can bring the pressure down by taking medication. Which solution would you say is best?

A New View of Health

But if health isn't feeling good, what *is* it? Can we look at health in a different way, one allowing us to get healthier, rather than only relieving symptoms? Yes, we can, and a good place to start is to look at the word "health".

If you were back in elementary school and your teacher asked for the root word of "health" you'd probably say, "heal". And you'd be right; a big part of health is your body's ability to heal itself.

For example, if you cut your finger and put a Band-Aid on it, does the Band-Aid heal the finger? Of course not. So there must be something **inside you** that knows how to heal the cut. The individual cells that are cut don't heal. They die. New cells are created to take their place. Most of what we call healing actually is the creation of new life.

Health is also how well your body functions. In other words, a person with a liver, heart, spleen, lungs, gall bladder, and every other organ functioning at 100 percent is much healthier than someone who has the same parts functioning at 60, 70 or 80 percent. So our new view of health must recognize that in order to get healthier we must get our bodies functioning better.

Health is not merely feeling good.
Health is your body's ability to heal, and function at a high level.
Chiropractic is all about helping your body do just that.

Health Is an Inside Job

Your liver performs more than 200 functions at various times throughout the day. Can you name them all? How about 50? Ten?

The doctor doesn't exist who can sit down and write from memory all the functions of the liver and every other organ. But there's one "doctor" who can. This doctor knows every function of every cell in your body. Do you know where to find this doctor? *Inside you.*

Doesn't it make sense that unless there was something inside of you controlling your liver, your liver wouldn't be working, because it's for sure that you aren't thinking about it. If you get eight hours of sleep tonight your heart will beat about 30,000 times. If you had to think about making your heart beat you wouldn't get much sleep.

We've been taught it's the pill, shot or surgery that heals. But life alone has the power to heal. Chiropractors are in the life business.

Like your liver and heart, right now every other part of your body is functioning at a certain level. How? What's in control? When I ask patients what part of their body controls all the other parts, the answer is unanimous: The brain.

Let's see how the brain is wired to every part of you, allowing it to control and coordinate your body's every function. Let's learn about, health-wise, the most important part of you, your *nervous system*.

2 THE WORLD'S GREATEST DOCTOR LIVES INSIDE OF YOU

[how your nervous system keeps you healthy]

You've Got A Lot of Nerve

The greatest doctor in the world is your nervous system. It's made of three parts. Your **brain** sits in your skull, protected on all sides by hard bone. Your **spinal cord** sits inside your spine. It extends from your brain to your low back. **Nerves** branch off from the cord and blaze millions of trails into your body, not stopping until they end right beneath your skin.

Your nervous system keeps your body running. As you read this sentence millions of **nerve impulses**--tiny electrical signals carrying information--are flashing back and forth over your nerves, as one part of your body communicates with others. While only a fraction as strong as a telephone signal, these electrical flashes let you think, make your muscles work and, through senses like sight and sound, tell you about the world outside yourself.

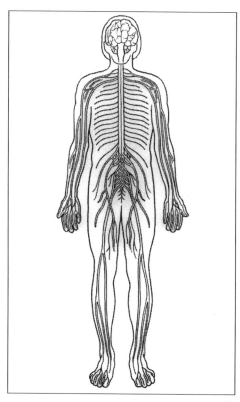

Top Gun

Right now your nervous system is keeping your heart beating, your lungs breathing and your hands holding this book. How do the different parts of your nervous system work to keep you thriving? Let's start at the top, with your brain, a creation that makes the latest, most powerful computer seem as technologically advanced as tinker toys. No one knows exactly how many brain cells are sitting between your ears, but estimates range from 10 billion to 100 billion.

Nerve cells talk to each other with electricity. A tiny electrical impulse travels from the center of one cell out over one of its branches. At the end of the branch there's a space about one millionth of an inch wide. The impulse jumps over this gap to a branch of the next cell.

"Every thought, every twitch of your finger, is an electrical event, or a series of electrical events," write Judith Hooper and Dick Teresi in their book on the brain, "The 3-Pound Universe":

"All the information that reaches you from the world…from the pattern of light and shadow that composes a face to the voice of the anchorman on the news…gets translated into a sequence of electrical pulses…"

Your brain is always lit up with electrical patterns forming, shifting, and dissolving, because the electrical link between nerve cells forms and vanishes in an instant.

But your brain isn't just a three-pound bag of nerve cells that think they're spark plugs. Groups of cells get together and form different sections of your brain, each performing a different job. Together, the parts of your brain form an incredibly powerful command post responsible for controlling and coordinating your body's every function.

As powerful as it is, without a way to speak with the rest of you, your brain would be a frustrated genius locked in a dark closet. That's why you have a spinal cord.

Life Line

Your spinal cord is a thick bundle of nerves. It exits from your skull and cascades down inside your spine, ending three to five inches above your waist. The vital messages traveling over it are carried out into your body by nerves branching off the cord.

Long Distance Direct

Your nerves are your body's telephone wires. As they exit the spinal cord they're packed into big bundles, like electrical cables. Then, almost immediately, they start branching out. As they travel farther from the spine they split into ever smaller threads, weaving their way through every inch of you. They are so numerous that if every part of you but your nerves disappeared, your friends could still recognize you because your nerves would form a 3-D image of incredible detail. While your nerves are like telephone wires, your body's nervous system is much more complex than any telephone network.

Control Freak

With your brain connected to your body through nerves you're equipped with a marvelous communication system. Nerves allow your brain to tell your big toe what to do. And if your big toe hits a bedpost in the middle of the night, it can very quickly tell your brain that it's unhappy.

There are many mysteries surrounding why and how the brain does what it does. One thing we do know is that many of the signals sent to control and coordinate your body take place in response to incoming information from your senses. Your brain changes your body in response to what you experience. Scientist call this your nervous system's ability to *adapt you to your environment.*

For example, let's say Mark gets a job as a ditch digger. His boss gives him a brand new shovel and says, "Go to it." Mark starts digging ditches eight hours a day.

At the end of a month, what would have happened to Mark's hands? They would be stronger and tougher. What about the shovel? It would have become dull and worn. Likewise, if you take aerobics classes your heart and muscles get stronger; but your shoes get worn. Your body gets stronger with use because your nervous system adapts you to stress.

Another amazing feature of this mind/body link is that **your brain can change your body in response to thoughts alone.**

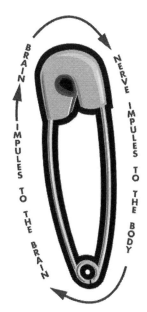

Let's say you're standing at the starting line, about to start a race. What will your heart be doing? Even though you're standing still, it will be beating fast, pumping blood through you like water through a fire hose. And this is happening **in anticipation** of the race.

The Safety Pin Cycle

The easiest way to think about how nerves connect your brain to your body is to imagine a safety pin. The pin has a top and bottom and is connected by two strands of wire. Your brain/body connection works the same way, with nerves flowing out from your brain into your body, and other nerves flowing from your body up to your brain. **When nerve impulses flow unobstructed around this loop, good health naturally flourishes, because the brain is controlling and coordinating your health with 100 percent efficiency.**

Intelligent Life in Your Universe

Where do we all come from? One cell from mama and one cell from papa. Think about that. Two cells you can't see with your naked eyes coming together and nine months later you get a beautiful little baby.

Do you think there is intelligence behind that process? Of course: If you ask a pregnant woman during the first few weeks of her pregnancy, "What are you making down there?" she won't be able to tell you. Yet there is a little person forming in her nonetheless, guided by an invisible life force.

What is the first thing formed in a new embryo? The spinal cord. Then the brain. And finally tiny little nerves branch off the cord. It's only after the central nervous system is formed that the rest of the organs take shape. The central nervous system is like the main computer, telling everything else what to become.

We've seen how there is something inside you that can heal a cut finger and raise your temperature when we're sick. This same intelligence creates a baby from two cells. This intelligence is carried in nerve impulses from your brain to every cell of your body, creating health inside you.

The founders of chiropractic realized that the key to health is the correct flow of intelligence over the body's nerves. This *inborn* or *innate intelligence* is in every living thing and is responsible for maintaining all living things in existence.

B.J. Palmer, the son of chiropractic's founder, D.D. Palmer, put it this way:

> *"Chiropractic teaches that the life principle, or Innate Intelligence, intelligently selects and assembles chemical elements found in human anatomy; it builds organs of the body for certain purposes, and then controls and governs their function and activities by means of these mental impulses created in the brain and sent over nerves to every tissue cell in the body.*
>
> *It is obvious that impairment of the brain or nerve tissue will interfere with the normal creation, transmission and expression of mental impulses, with the result that the cells which these nerves supply will not receive or express the proper command; will not coordinate or work in harmony with the rest of the organism, and then we have a condition of disease, or lack of ease."*

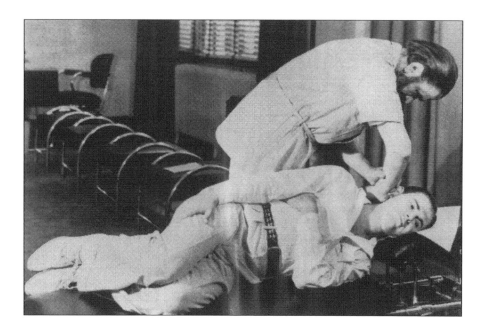

"The physical organism, your body, has its own intelligence, as does the organism of every other life-form...The body's intelligence is, of course, an inseparable part of universal intelligence, one of its countless manifestations. It gives temporary cohesion to the atoms and molecules that make up your physical organism. It is the organizing principle behind the workings of all the organs of the body, the conversion of oxygen and food into energy, the heartbeat and circulation of the blood, the immune system that protects the body from invaders, the translation of sensory input into nerve impulses that are sent to the brain, decoded there, and reassembled into a coherent inner picture of reality. All these, as well as thousands of other simultaneously occurring functions, are coordinated perfectly by that intelligence. You don't run your body. The intelligence does..."

Housing Crisis

In studying the nervous system chiropractors asked, "How can this wonderful system we're equipped with, whereby the brain controls the body using nerves, develop problems?"

They found the answer in the spine.

In your body your brain is protected by hard bone, your skull. Just as the skull protects the brain, the spine protects the spinal cord. Instead of being solid, however, the spine is made up of 24 bones stacked on top of each other like ABC blocks. In order to allow us to bend and twist the 24 spinal bones move. And because they move, they can and do get out of alignment. When bones become misaligned they put pressure on the nerves exiting the spine, pinching and irritating them, causing problems.

What happens when nerves become pinched? Let's see. . .

3 THE WORLD'S GREATEST DOCTOR IS OVERLOADED

[how stress creates subluxations]

B.J. Palmer giving a chiropractic adjustment at his research clinic.

True Lies

Miracles are happening in chiropractic offices every day. 12-year-olds who've been wetting the bed for years stop after two visits to their chiropractor. People suffering with migraine headaches all their lives are headache-free after the top bone of their neck is properly aligned. Sinus problems clear up. Chronic rashes heal. Eyesight improves. Asthma conditions go away. Chronic back pain becomes a thing of the past within a week or two of care.

How? How can one person be relieved of headaches, another of bedwetting, a third made to see better, and a fourth have her skin clear up, because a chiropractor has improved the functioning of their nervous systems?

The answer is that chiropractors don't treat heads, bladders, eyes, or skin. By relieving nerve pressure, they release the ability of their patients' bodies to heal all these ailments and many more. They set free the intelligence carried in the nerve impulses flowing from the brain to the body and from the body up to the brain. When they do this, the body heals itself.

21

Block Party

What happens to create misaligned vertebrae and the resulting nerve pressure in the first place? In a word: stress. Physical, emotional, mental or chemical stress causes the normal alignment of our spines to become distorted.

These spinal misalignments are called **subluxations**. A subluxation is a bone out of place in the spine, irritating nerves and causing our bodies to function incorrectly. Subluxations formed when your nervous system is overwhelmed by physical stress are the easiest to understand.

For example, let's say you're in a whiplash-type car accident. The impact's force knocks the bones in your neck out of their normal alignment. When neck bones get knocked out of position they pinch, or put pressure on, the nerves exiting from the neck vertebrae. Now, wherever these nerves are traveling to in the body experiences a loss of function.

If the subluxations aren't corrected, other problems result. Because the bones are out of alignment, they start wearing and grinding down the joints and discs around them. This abnormal alignment leads to arthritis and degenerative joint disease. It's like a wobbly tire on a car: It's going to wear out faster. The muscles attaching into these misplaced vertebrae never work the same, either. They remain tight and tense, or abnormally loose.

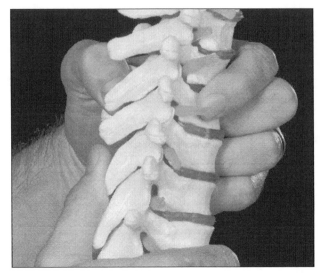

Normal spinal alignment: Note the large opening for the nerve to exit the spine.

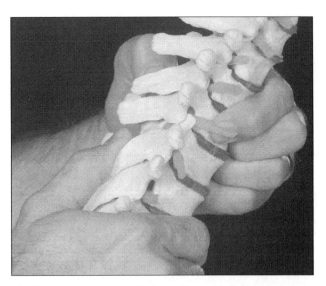

As bones move out of place they close the opening where nerves exit the spine, putting pressure on the nerves.

Entry-Level Conditions

Injuries resulting from a car accident are easy to understand. Other traumas may not be so apparent. For example, the very first physical trauma many of us experience is being born. A normal birth would be the mother pushing the baby out with the assistance of gravity. But in our society many times babies are delivered from the birth canal by physicians that twist and pull the baby out. Some common health conditions associated with subluxations that occur at birth are colic, chronic ear infections, respiratory problems such as asthma, frequent colds, allergies, headaches and neck pain.

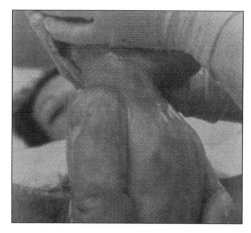

Twist and shout.
The birth process may cause pinched nerves in the neck.

One of the most exciting recent developments in chiropractic is the growing trend of parents bringing their children to the chiropractor for regular check-ups. And it's interesting to note: very few two and three-year-olds come into the chiropractor's office in pain. With the exception of headaches and traumas ("Tommy was jumping on the trampoline and landed on Karen's head. Can I bring them in?"), their subluxations aren't causing pain, yet their bodies are not working correctly. When we relieve the pressure on their nerves, our children's bodies work better.

Bad Chemistry

Chemical stresses can cause subluxations, too. Studies have shown that certain chemicals, including drugs, food additives, tobacco smoke and air pollution can also cause irritated, tight muscles, leading to subluxations. Mental stress affects our bodies the same way. If we always feel anxious, our muscles become tight and tense. If we keep tightening our muscles in response to mental stress, bones get pulled out of position (see page 27, "The Hidden Cause of Subluxations").

Thus, subluxations can occur whenever your body encounters a physical, chemical or "mentallemotional" health stress that is greater than your body's natural resistance.

In A Pinch

An easy way to think about subluxations is to imagine water flowing through a hose. If you're watering flowers with a hose and someone steps on it, what happens to the flow of water? If the flowers don't get water, they develop problems. If areas of our bodies don't receive proper nerve flow, they develop problems, too.

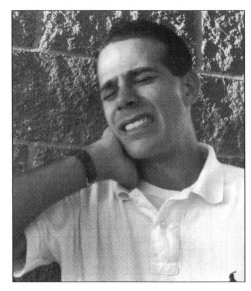

Pressure gauge: Neck pain often results from pinched nerves.

Studies show that even a small pressure on spinal nerves causes a drastic decrease in their ability to work. For example, at the University of Colorado, a researcher focusing on how the spine works devised the following experiment: Cats were given back surgeries. Nerves exiting the spine were hooked to instruments measuring their function. Weights were then placed on the nerves to see how much function was lost. With the weight of a dime on it, a spinal nerve lost up to 60 percent of its normal nerve flow. What effect do you think that would have on the organs that nerve was supplying with nerve impulses?

Other studies have demonstrated what happens to the human body when subluxations decrease nerve supply. Dr. Henry Winsor, a medical doctor, was inspired by chiropractic literature to experiment and see if there was a relationship between subluxations and organ disease. In a series of three studies done at the University of Pennsylvania, he dissected 75 human and 22 cat cadavers. Of 221 organs found to be diseased, 212 were supplied by nerves that were being pinched by spinal subluxations. For example, all 26 cadavers showing lung disease had subluxations in the upper back, where the nerves sending messages to the lungs exit the spine.

The field of somato-visceral disease (the study of how the body's structure affects organ function) is booming today, proving what chiropractors have been saying for more than a hundred years.

As Time Goes By

Many patients walking into a chiropractor's office are bringing in subluxations they've had since childhood, even birth. All that time their bodies may have been pain-free, even while working at less than 100 percent. But over time the body reaches a point where symptoms develop.

An example would be an office worker with painful wrists and hands. She may have been told she has "carpel tunnel syndrome," a condition in which the hands, wrists and forearms can become extremely painful.

Typically, the first symptom these patients notice is wrist and finger pain. Then, after several months, numbness in the hands. Soon these become mixed with sharp, shooting pains into the forearms. The pain might even wake the person at night. Many times such patients have a history of neck trauma, such as whiplash-type car accidents. The injury creates subluxations in the neck, where nerves come out and run to the arms and fingers. When nerve flow is obstructed the wrists lose their ability to work correctly. Over time, bones in the wrists become misaligned and pinch nerves in the area. While the symptoms are in the wrists, the main problem is the subluxations in the neck that have been there for years.

Old Times

Subluxations cause problems other than a loss of function and pain. For example, clench your hand into a tight fist. Can you feel how much more energy tight muscles use than those that are relaxed? Subluxations are often accompanied by tight, spasmed muscles, as your body strains to correct its alignment. As such, subluxations are energy sinkholes, gobbling up vitality we could use in other areas of life. One of my favorite chiropractic quotes isn't from a chiropractor. It's from Dr. Robert Sperry, the 1980 Nobel Prize winner for brain research. Dr. Sperry noted that, "The more mechanically misaligned someone is, the less energy they will have for thinking, metabolism and healing."

Besides draining energy, subluxations make us old before our time. Your biological age is simply a measure of how well your body works, compared to time. For example, a 50-year-old marathon runner might have the heart of a 20-year-old but the knees of a 57-year-old. A key factor in figuring biological age is *flexibility*. A loss of flexibility accompanies any misalignment in the body. As your bones shift out of their normal position they stop moving correctly. The bones often jam and begin sending out pain signals that cause muscle spasms in the area. Every day in practice I see long-time chiropractic patients in their forties and fifties with more flexible spines than new patients in their twenties and thirties. They may be older, but in some important respects they're actually younger.

Along with everything else, subluxations bring us down mentally and emotionally, because if your body isn't performing well, it's hard to think clearly or stay positive. *In truth, every aspect of your being--from your energy supply to your mental clarity to your outlook on life--is affected by subluxations in your spine.*

Do You Have Spinal Problems?

Top Ten Warning Signs

1. You can turn your head further to one side than the other. For example, you can turn your head to the right so that your chin is nearly over your shoulder, but when you turn to the left your head gets "stuck" well before your shoulder. This indicates vertebrae in the neck are out of alignment.

2. You feel as if the muscles at the base of your neck are always tight and tense. This indicates a long-standing postural distortion, where your muscles are straining to keep your head in proper alignment.

3. When you look at the heels of your shoes, they show a different wear pattern. For example, one heel might be worn more on the back outside edge. Uneven wear patterns indicate an imbalance in your hips, knees or feet.

4. You frequently get colds and flues (more than once a year). This indicates lowered immunity, often brought on by spinal subluxations affecting your immune system.

5. You wake up in the morning with low back pain. This is usually the result of misalignments of your lumbar, or lower back, vertebrae.

6. You have poor posture, with your shoulders rounded and your head carried in front of your shoulders. A "slumped" posture indicates spinal misalignments.

7. Your foot (or feet) flares out to the side when you walk. Take a walk, and look down at your feet as you stride. Do the toes point straight ahead, or does one or both of your feet point out to the side when you walk? If so, this indicates hip problems, which add stress to your low back as well.

8. You frequently "crack" your neck or back. Tension builds in these subluxated areas, and twisting your neck or back until you hear a pop relieves this built-up tension. But you are usually moving hyper mobile joints (ones moving *too* much) while the real culprits stay stuck. You aren't fixing the real problem, and as the tension returns you feel you must pop your neck or back again.

9. You are always tired. It takes a lot more energy to live with a body that is not properly aligned. Most people report more energy under chiropractic care, because the energy that used to be "bound up" in the spine is freed for more useful purposes.

10. Your jaw makes popping and clicking noises. Often times the jaw joints (also known as the temporomandibular joints--TMJ's) become misaligned. This problem can also be caused by misalignments in the neck. Fortunately, many TMJ problems respond wonderfully to chiropractic adjustments.

The "Hidden" Cause of Subluxations

It's easy to see how falling down the stairs or sustaining a whiplash injury could knock bones out of alignment in the spine. But any chiropractor whose been practicing for awhile will tell you emotional and mental stresses can cause subluxations, too.

Think about the last time you were really angry. Do you remember how tight the muscles in your jaw, neck and shoulders felt? Tight muscles can pull bones out of alignment.

Mental stress affects our bodies the same way. If we keep tightening our muscles in response to mental stress, bones get pulled out of position. Later you'll learn how to use your brain to help keep your spine in alignment.

Blind Sight

Right now you may be asking yourself, "Why haven't I ever heard any of this from my medical doctor?" Good question! The fact is that most medical doctors have never been to a chiropractor, never talked to a chiropractor, and, if they have been exposed to the subject of chiropractic in their schooling, have heard all the negative myths earlier generations of doctors were led to believe out of ignorance.

If you've read this book up to this point you know more about chiropractic than most medical doctors. This sounds absurd, but it's true. So don't be surprised if your medical doctor doesn't diagnose your subluxations.

Reeling from the Years

Physical, emotional, mental, and chemical stresses can produce subluxations. By creating parts of us that are inflexible and rigid, where life doesn't flow, subluxations deaden us. As time goes on, they accumulate in our bodies. We take them on as baggage as we go through life, so that by the time we reach our 20's or 30's (or 60's or 70s), large parts of our bodies are functioning at less than maximum potential.

In the rest of this book you'll learn about how chiropractic can help you regain your ability to heal and function at the highest level possible, and how it can help you achieve optimal health.

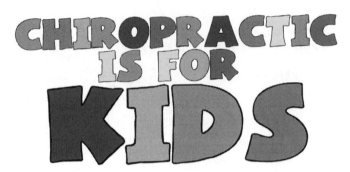

More and more parents are bringing their children to the chiropractor for regular check-ups. "Johnny doesn't have any back or neck pains. Why would I bring him to a chiropractor?" you might ask.

Think about this: You take your children to the dentist to get their teeth checked. You have their eyes and hearing checked. Doesn't it make sense to have their spines checked as well? Remember, the nerves exiting the spine are the lifelines between your children's brains and their bodies. If there is interference in the lifeline, problems will eventually develop. Like cavities in teeth, these problems can be corrected if detected early enough.

Chiropractic kids are healthier kids! And with their spines in line your children will need fewer drugs, with their often dangerous side effects.

If your child has never been checked for subluxations they need to be, especially if they have any of the following conditions:	
▪ Eye problems	▪ ADHD Disorders
▪ Frequent stomach aches	▪ Persistent cough
▪ Neurological conditions	▪ Poor posture, including foot flare
▪ Neck or back pain	▪ Scoliosis (curvature of the spine)
▪ Pain in the shoulders, arms, hands	▪ Sinus/allergy problems
▪ Hip, knee or foot pain	▪ Nervousness, difficulty concentrating
▪ Asthma	▪ Headaches
▪ Bedwetting	▪ Constipation
▪ Colic	▪ Ear Infections

4 POSING PROBLEMS

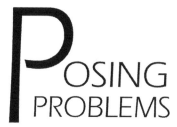

[posture's dramatic impact on your health]

Curves Ahead

"Stand up straight!" mothers beg their slumping children, and for good reason. Posture affects our appearance and health in remarkable ways.

For example, David was a teenager whose mother brought him to a chiropractor because of neck and back pain. David had always been sickly, spending several weeks each year hospitalized with pneumonia. Each day he swallowed blood pressure medication, though his doctors were at a loss to explain why his blood pressure remained high.

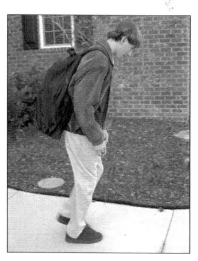

WARNING: Poor posture can start early in life.

An x-ray of this fifteen-year-old's back showed his spine dramatically curved to the side, a condition known as scoliosis. Scoliosis causes many postural problems, ranging from uneven hips and shoulders to a "hunchback".

David's spine was curved most in the upper back, where nerves exit and travel to the lungs and heart. His chiropractor felt that many of his health problems stemmed from pinched nerves along his spine, and told him that along with getting rid of his back pain, there was a good chance he could keep him out of the hospital. He didn't mention chiropractic's success at lowering blood pressure in many patients.

David progressed rapidly, his pain fading in about two weeks. During his third week of care he visited his "blood pressure doctor". Remarkably, his blood pressure had dropped a full ten points! He continued to improve, and now he's medication-free and his lungs are working fine. This is a surprisingly common example of a patient's posture compromising heart and lung function.

In order for you to "stand up straight," you need a spine with four front-to-back curves. Your neck and low back curve forward, your middle spine and tailbone curve back.

Your spine's curves keep you functioning in the fast lane. Your neck and low back's forward curves help support your head squarely over your shoulders and your torso over your hips. The middle of your back slopes backward to make room for your heart and lugs. Likewise your tailbone, also curving back, gives your bladder and colon room to fill, and in women it eases a baby's trip from the womb.

Stooped and Conquered

The most common posture problem is when a person loses the natural curve in their neck and their head drops forward. This can be caused by trauma such as whiplash-type injuries. It can also happen over time when we constantly bend forward to read, work at a desk, watch television and eat. In fact, most of us spend our lives bending toward the front of our bodies to one degree or another. Over time, our posture can change as our heads drop in front of our shoulders. At the extreme, this is the classic "old lady" posture, where the person's entire body is bent forward. The average head weighs 8-12 pounds. As it drops down it's no longer supported easily over the shoulders. Instead, the neck muscles must strain to keep the head up.

It's now known that a forward-bent head posture is at the root cause of many health problems. One reason is that as the head drops, the neck's natural curve is lost and the spinal cord is abnormally stretched. This tension changes the way your nervous system processes information: Your whole body can be "thrown off" because of this postural distortion.

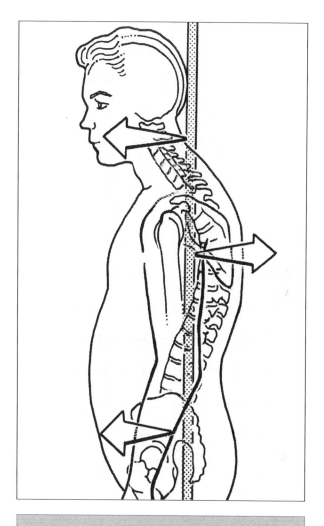

This is the most typical postural distortion. The head is dropped forward, and there is an increased mid-and upper back curve as the shoulders slump forward. The pelvis is rocked forward, and the feet are "pronated," with a loss of their normal arch and more weight placed on the inside of their arches.

With this posture, tension and stress accumulates in the spinal cord and muscles throughout the body, especially at the base of the neck.

Family Posture Check-up

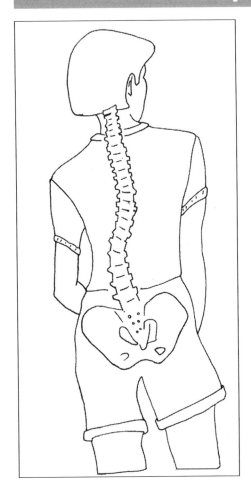

- [ ] The person being checked should stand looking straight ahead, arms to their sides, in a neutral position.
- [ ] Stand behind the person being checked.
- [ ] Place the fingertips of your left hand under the person's left ear; the fingertips of your right hand under their right ear.
- [ ] Check the level of the person's ears and mark your findings below.
- [ ] Place your hands on the shoulders. Note if the shoulders are level.
- [ ] Place your hands on the top of the hips. They should be level with the floor.
- [ ] If you note a high ear, shoulder or hip your family member or friend should be checked by a chiropractor immediately.

Head Left Right _____	Head. Ears Level	Head - tilted. One ear slightly higher.	Head - tilted. One ear markedly higher.
Shoulders Left Right _____	Shoulders level. (Horizontally)	One Shoulder. Slightly higher than the other.	One Shoulder. Markedly higher than the other.
Hips Left Right _____	Hips level. (Horizontally)	One Hip. Slightly higher.	One Hip. Markedly higher.

In a Pinch

Poor posture is at the root of many headache problems. How? Because when neck muscles tighten inappropriately, they can tug the first and second bones of the neck out of their normal positions. As the bones become misaligned, they put pressure on nearby nerves, which are responsible for controlling the function of blood vessels and muscles on the scalp.

Soon scalp muscles spasm and blood vessels constrict. Often the headaches created by pinched nerves start at the base of the skull, intensifying as they move onto the head and wrap around to the temples. Chiropractic "cures" these headaches by relieving nerve pressure so muscles and blood vessels can function normally.

Tension Headaches

Tension headaches are very common, affecting forty percent of teenagers and adults. At the root cause of most tension headaches, which usually start in the neck or at the back of the head, are misaligned vertebrae.

As we've seen, once bones become misaligned, they put pressure on nerves exiting the spine and running throughout the body. Once bones in the neck get out of alignment, they put pressure on the nerves traveling to the back of the neck and up onto the head. The pinched nerves cause muscles and blood vessels in the neck and scalp to tighten, causing the "vise like" feeling many people report with tension headaches. (Incidentally, this is why stress triggers tension headaches: When you are under stress the muscles in your neck tighten, which can pull misaligned bones even farther out of place, putting more pressure on nerves.)

Nine major university studies found that chiropractic adjustments were better than medication at helping patients with tension headaches—without the drugs' side effects.

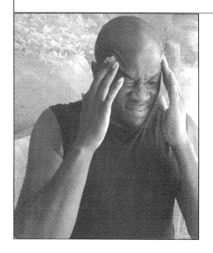

Do You Suffer From Tension Headaches?

At the back of this book you'll find a "Special Help" section for headaches that gives you tips and tools to help with this common health problem. *You'll find information on:*

- How relaxation techniques help with headaches.
- Foods to avoid if you suffer from headaches.
- How you can use magnesium and peppermint to stop headache pain.

Time Bombs

Poor posture can also cause a spasm-pain-spasm cycle in the neck. When neck muscles stay tense, small pockets of extremely tight muscles develop, called "trigger points". Trigger points are dime-sized land mines waiting to explode in the neck and head. When tense muscles are stressed, trigger points within them activate. This throws the muscle tissue surrounding the point into painful spasm. Pain signals race to the brain, and the brain, in a protective reflex, increases muscle tension *even more*.

Some of the most hazardous trigger points are the ones located right beneath the skull. As these fire, muscles on the head and neck spasm, creating headaches. When examining a patient suffering from chronic headaches I often find pinched nerves and trigger points in an area right beneath the back of the skull. (See the "Trigger Fingers" exercise in this chapter's "Neck Pain Relief" program.)

Breath Control

Posture problems can also drain our energy by robbing our oxygen supply. *Do this test:* Drop your head and shoulders forward in a slump, so your chin rests on or near your chest. Try taking a deep breath through your nose. Notice how noisy the breath is and how the air going into your lungs stops at the top of your chest. Now hold your head up and your shoulders back. Take another breath. Can you feel how the air streams in more easily, flowing freely toward the bottom of your ribcage?

Muscle Bound

When your spine becomes misaligned, your muscles do their best to pull you back into shape. They tense, they tighten, and like Winston Churchill in his famous line, they never, never, never quit. Most patients walk into my office carrying backs riddled with extremely tight, painful muscles straining to realign their spines.

For example, often when examining a patient's hips I will find one hip positioned higher than the other. Because our legs attach to our hips, every time these patients take a step they put more weight on one side of their bodies. Over time, the resulting muscle imbalance will cause pain and tension in the muscles between the shoulder blades and upper back.

Same Old Grind

Joints are affected by poor posture, too. A smooth, shock-absorbing material called cartilage covers the ends of bones and keeps them from grinding against each other. If bones remain aligned, their cartilage-covered ends move as smoothly as marbles rolling on a polished floor.

If bones lose their proper alignment, their cartilage-covered ends begin grinding. Inflammation sets in, and soon the cartilage starts breaking down. Ultimately, misalignments lead to one of the most common health problems of our time, degenerative arthritis.

"Arthritis" simply means "inflammation of a joint" (from the Latin, in which "arthra" means "joint" and "itis" means "inflammation"). Unfortunately, most physicians do not recognize the role of misalignments in causing arthritis or that restoring proper alignment may dramatically improve the condition.

Bone Tired

It's not just cartilage that wears out when your spine becomes misaligned. Bones degenerate, too. Perhaps the best examples are misalignments created by whiplash-type auto accident injuries.

In a classic whiplash the car is hit from behind. As the car jolts forward, its passengers' heads snap back. Then the car suddenly stops and their heads snap forward. It's estimated that about 30 percent of all drivers will suffer a whiplash during their lives.

The Powerful Forces of Whiplash

During a whiplash your head's weight (8 to 12 pounds) becomes a powerful force. Typically, as you are hit from behind, your head is whipped backwards past its normal range of motion. As it does, muscles and ligaments tear and disks and joints become injured. As your car jerks to a stop your head whips forward. Even more injury occurs. Your neck may now curve backward instead of forward. You now have a recipe for pain: The torn and injured muscles, ligaments, discs, and joints become swollen and painful, yet now must support the full weight of you head.

1) Before impact, your neck's natural curve is aligned.

2) Your head whips backward, exaggerating your neck's curve.

3) Your head snaps forward, reversing your neck's natural curve.

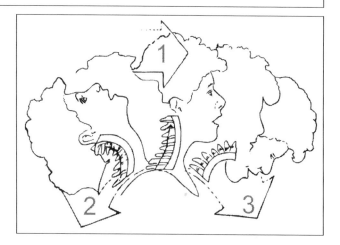

Whiplash injuries produce misalignments throughout the body, but most damage occurs in the neck, which often loses its natural curve. Now when the person twists, bends or turns these normal movements are forced upon misaligned bones. Often the bones start pinching nerves and the person develops headaches, neck pain, and tingling and numbness in the arms and fingers. Inflammation also develops and the slow process of degeneration begins, leading to arthritis.

Here is a typical example: A 37-year-old man comes into the chiropractic office complaining of sharp, intense neck pain that shoots down his shoulders and into his arms. He reports that he was in a "real bad" motorcycle accident as a teenager; he has been living with neck pain for 15 years. On X-ray, there is a tidal wave of degenerative arthritis in his neck. Its fourth, fifth and sixth bones have degenerated so badly they have developed bone "spurs". These are small horn-shaped bits of bone that eventually grow together and fuse the spine into a rigid, cement-like structure. It's thought they are the body's method of stabilizing areas of the spine where degeneration changes normal movement.

Most people try to handle arthritis pain with over-the-counter and prescription pain relievers. Unfortunately, blocking the pain signals from degenerating joints does nothing to restore their health, and actually harms several organ systems in your body.

The Price You Pay for "Over the Counter" Pain Relief

Aspirin (Bayer, Bufferin, Ecotrin): Causes stomach bleeding; overuse can lead to ulcers. Aspirin, Ibuprofen and Naproxen send over 100,000 people to the hospital each year with ulcers and other gastrointestinal disorders.

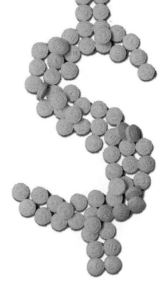

Ibuprofen (Advil, Motrin, Nuprin): Damages the stomach lining, puts abnormal stress on the kidney and liver.

Naproxen (Aleve): Linked to increased heart disease, damages stomach lining, puts abnormal stress on the kidney and liver.

Acetaminophen (Tylenol, Aspirin-Free Anacin): Puts abnormal stress on the liver. Acetaminophen is responsible for nearly half of all cases of acute liver failure.

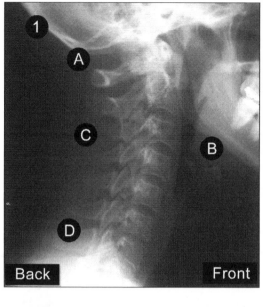

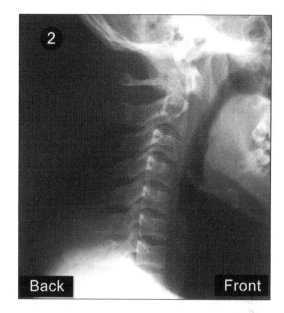

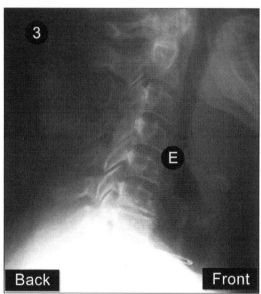

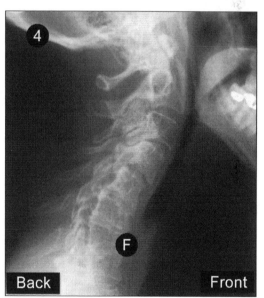

Reversed aging. These x-rays are side-views of the neck's seven vertebrae. To orient yourself: A is at the back of your skull. B: bottom of the jaw. C: back of the neck. D: base of the neck, where it joins the shoulders. The neck should curve forward (1). Trauma or other stress can cause the neck's normal curve to reverse (2). Now bones degenerate, losing their normal square shape as bone "spurs" develop (3/E). As degeneration continues, bones fuse together (4/F).

Why Chiropractors Adjust Their Patients

When you go to a Chiropractor as a patient you will be *adjusted*. "What is that?" you might ask.

Chiropractors *adjust* misaligned bones—subluxations--back into place. Using a variety of techniques, they re-train your body back into proper alignment. Here's why:

If you are getting the proper nutrition, then all the ingredients you need to stay healthy are in your body. From the moment of birth your body uses what you eat and drink to make its own insulin, adrenalin, pepsin, hydrochloric acid, enzymes, blood, sweat, tears, and thousands of other chemicals.

So when you cut yourself, your skin heals from the inside, with materials made by your body. If you break a bone, it heals from the inside, using materials you make inside yourself. Your body heals itself, and this healing is directed by your nervous system.

But you aren't just a chemical factory, you're also a marvelous machine. Your body is a mechanical structure made up of hundreds of moving parts. There are more than two hundred bones in the body. The spinal bones are special. They move freely so you can bend and twist. But because they are freely movable, they can get out of adjustment. Ask any engineer or mechanic about a machine with moving parts. He will tell you that no machine can operate twenty-four hours a day, month after month and year after year, without getting out of adjustment.

As you go through life you run, jump and fall. You heave, strain, lug and tug. You get jarred, jolted and bruised, all of which can work the bones of your body out of adjustment. And when they get out of adjustment these bones irritate the nerves controlling all the different functions in your body. The parts of your body served by these nerves are deprived of their normal nerve flow...and they get sick.

To restore health, normal nerve function must be restored. To restore normal nerve function, the structural parts of your body that have been strained or jolted out of position must be adjusted back into place. When this is done they no longer block or irritate nerves. Then the nervous system can again direct the normal processes of your body, and if damage has not gone too far, the body can heal.

Drugs can't adjust you back to normal.

You were born with a complete chemical factory. But you weren't born with complete mechanical equipment. At birth you couldn't even crawl, much less walk, balance, run and jump. As you grew you adapted to all the stresses of life, and you got out of adjustment.

That's why Chiropractors adjust their patients.

Pain and Posture Relief

What makes your neck hurt? The answer is pinched nerves and tight muscles. Once a nerve is pinched and muscles in the area tighten and stay tight, several things happen that lead to pain.

One, the muscles begin working much harder than normal. You saw this before when you clinched your fist and felt how hard your muscles work when they are tight. But that's not the only problem. All that effort produces chemical waste in the muscles. If you hold your fist clenched for a period of time you will notice the blood drains out of it. That is because as the muscles tighten they squeeze blood from the arteries, capillaries and veins in the area. Now you have created a recipe for pain: The muscles are tight, producing waste, but there is not enough blood flow to wash the waste away.

Sometimes we develop tight areas in our bodies, but they are not tight enough to produce discomfort. Then we get stressed, and the added stress creates enough additional muscle tension to produce pain. When you relax, the pain stops, but that area of your body remains tight and tense, waiting to produce more pain the next time you are stressed.

Exercises for the neck and back help relieve pain by loosening the muscles, allowing more blood to flow through them, eliminating the waste products of muscular effort and allowing misaligned bones to gain better alignment.

The following **Neck Pain Relief** exercises aim to relieve stress in the neck and shoulders, the areas most prone to problems caused by poor posture. If you are suffering from headaches or pain/tension in the neck and shoulders, concentrate on this easy 10-minute routine. For best results do it twice a day, morning and evening. If you're limited on time it's best to do the exercises in the morning, after taking a warm shower. You can also do the Self Massage portion of the routine throughout the day. Once you are out of pain, pick two or three of the exercises from the routine to do daily. This will keep your muscles loose.

Breathe Right / Stretch Better

Throughout this book you'll find great stretches to keep your body flexible and aligned. You'll get more benefit from stretching if you breathe correctly. Your breath has two phases: The "in" breath, which is the energizing phase, and the "out" breath, which is the relaxation phase. Your body naturally relaxes as you let a breath out. So it's usually best to breathe out as you stretch your muscles to new lengths. Also, unless otherwise noted, take long, slow, deep breaths, breathing in though your nose, and out through your mouth.

Neck Pain Relief
Approximate workout time: 10 minutes

Basic Neck Stretch

You can do this stretch anywhere, but it works particularly well in the shower, when you can let warm water flow against the muscles being stretched:

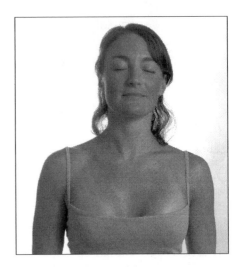

- Sit or stand up straight. Pretend there's a big hot air balloon directly overhead, and it's pulling your head straight up into the air. Feel your muscles stretch. Every time you breathe out lift your head up toward the ceiling or sky even more.

- Now retract your chin back toward your neck. This is not the same as tucking your chin. Your jaw should remain parallel with the floor as you bring your neck back and make a "double chin".

- Now, exhale slowly and let your neck drop to the side, so that your ear approximates your shoulder. Don't push your head down toward your shoulder; let the weight of your head do the stretching.

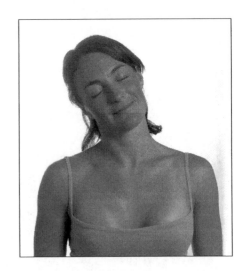

- Keep your head stretched and take two more breaths in and out, each time letting the weight of your head bring your ear closer to your shoulder, getting a good stretch on the opposite side of your neck.

- Repeat to the opposite side.

Basic Neck Stretch Using Chair

This is a particularly good stretch for those with pain running from their neck into the tops of their shoulders. You do it while sitting in a firm, straight-backed chair.

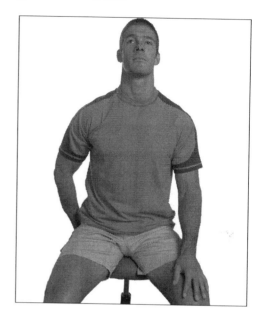

- Sit up straight, with your feet flat on the floor. With your right hand take hold of the chair so that you are holding onto it behind your right hip joint. (You may have to move to the front of your chair to accomplish this.)

- Imagine there is a big hot air balloon pulling your head straight up toward the sky.

- Retract your chin.

- Now let your breath out and let your head and torso drop forward, away from your anchored arm. Let yourself drop all the way forward, as far as your arm will allow.

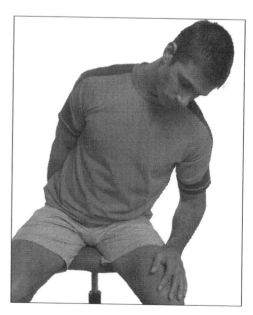

- Stretch for three complete breaths, dropping forward every time you let a breath out.

- Repeat to the opposite side.

Note: Once your head and torso are dropped forward, turn your chin gently a few degrees from side to side. You'll notice different areas of your shoulder muscles being stretched, and can isolate the ones that are tightest. Once you do, hold your chin in the position that gives that part of your shoulder the best stretch.

The Shoulder Shrug

*Many people instinctively shrug their shoulders to relieve tension in this area. The keys to making shoulder shrugs work for you are to do them **slowly**, with **proper breathing**. Here is how:*

- Stand or sit up straight. Taking a long, slow, deep breath into your belly, begin to raise your shoulders. Continue breathing in as your shoulders come up as high as they can stretch, and keep breathing as you push the shoulders back.

- When your shoulders are pushed as far up and back as they will comfortably stretch, begin to breathe out. As you slowly let your breath out, push your shoulders down and then forward and up.

- As you begin to breathe in again repeat the up-and-back movements, breathing out as you push the shoulders down and forward. Exaggerate the movements as much as possible without causing yourself pain. Don't speed up. The slower the better.

- Do four repetitions.

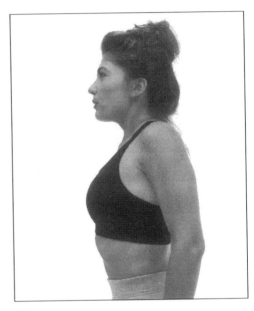

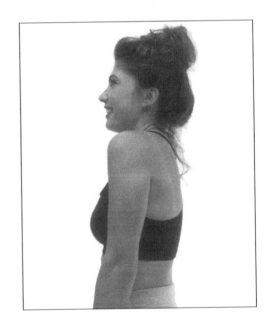

Shoulder Shrug Two

Now that your shoulders and neck are warmed up it's time to increase your stretching movements:

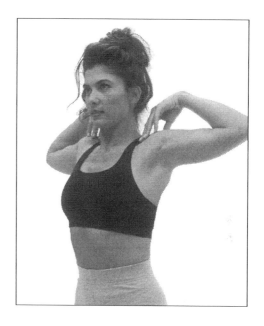

- Place your fingertips on your shoulders. As you breathe in, raise your elbows up and back; as you breathe out bring the elbows down as far toward the ground as possible, lifting them up and forward so that your elbows come together in front of your chest.

- Note: Your breath should be let out all the way as your elbows meet in front of your chest.

- Begin breathing in again as you bring the elbows back up toward the ceiling, out to the sides and back.

- Repeat four times.

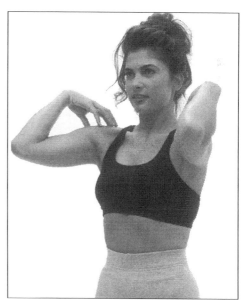

The Reader

■ Start by holding your hands in front of you, palms shoulder height and facing you as if you were reading a book.

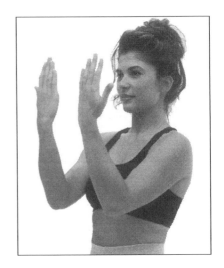

■ As you breathe in deeply, raise your arms and keep your eyes on your "book" so that your head arches back. Don't arch your back. You should feel a good stretch under your arms and across your chest. With your arms stretched, hold the pose and your breath for a count of two.

■ Now exhale fully and slowly drop your head toward your chest, letting your head hang limp as you exhale fully.

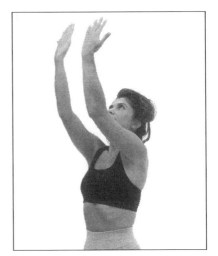

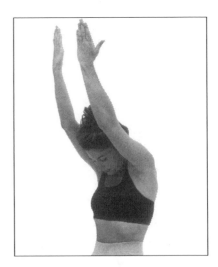

* Take another breath in and, keeping your arms in an L-shape, press your elbows back so that your chest fully stretches and expands. Hold for a count of two.

* Now breathe out and pretend you're diving off a diving board, bringing both arms as far out in front of your body as you can while letting your head drop to your chest. Hold for a count of two.

* Inhaling, come back to the starting position.

* Exhale and let your chin drop to your chest.

* Inhale. Lift your head so that you are "reading" your book, and start again.

* Repeat four times.

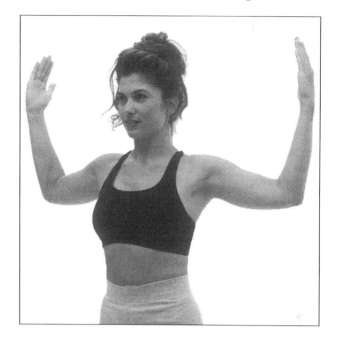

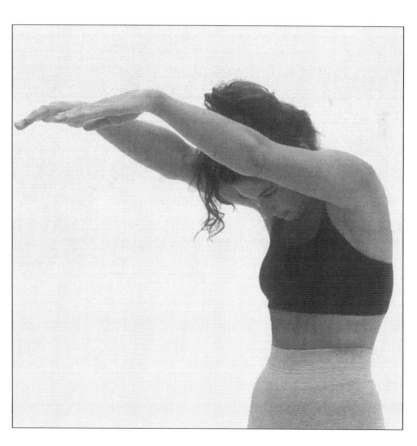

Trigger Fingers

The explosive trigger points in your neck and skull muscles that are at the root of so many "tension" headaches can be defused with this exercise.

- Start by lying on your back. Get comfortable. Turn your head to the left. Using your thumb, press into the base of your skull, just behind your right ear. If it's sore/tender, it's probably a trigger point. Press firmly into the spot. This will cause some pain; don't overdo it. Hold for a full count of seven, counting "one-thousand one, one-thousand two, etc." Release.

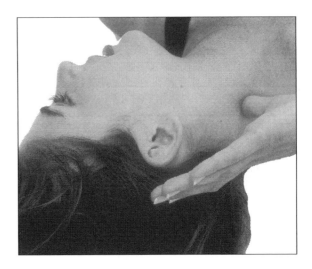

- Now move one thumbs-width in toward the center of your skull and again press in. If this spot is sore, press for seven seconds. If not, move one thumb's-width in again toward the center of your skull and press again. Keep pressing along the groove right beneath your skull, finding trigger points and pressing into them for seven seconds.

- Move along toward the middle of your skull, erasing trigger points as you go. When you reach the center of your skull, turn your head to the right and do the left side.

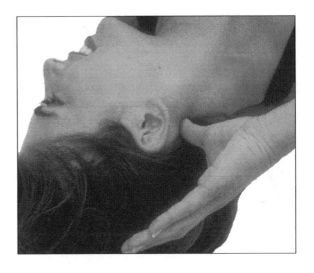

Note: Do the Trigger Fingers exercise twice each day while lying in bed, in the morning when you first wake up and at night when you go to bed. You should notice that some of the tender points become less tender, and may even disappear. The ones that are left are often the ones that trigger your headaches/neck pain. Once you know them, you can often prevent headaches or neck pain by working on them at the first sign of trouble.

Trigger Fingers With A Partner

A partner can be very helpful when working on trigger points in the neck and shoulders. Here's how to work with a partner to rid your body of these "pains in the neck":

- The person getting worked on (we'll call them the "patient") should sit comfortably in a chair. The person doing the trigger point work (we'll call them the "partner") stands at their left side, and places the palm of their left hand on the patient's forehead. The patient let's their head drop forward, letting their neck and shoulders relax.

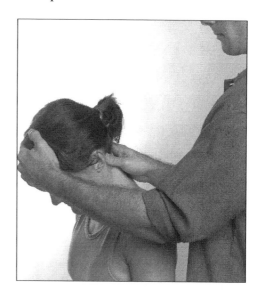

- While supporting the patient's head, the partner takes the thumb of their right hand and places it on the skull of the patient, right behind the left ear (see photo). Now, with their thumb at a 45 degree angle, the partner slides their thumb down into the groove right beneath the skull, pushes into the muscles and asks, "Is that sore?" It's up to the patient to tell the partner if they've hit a sore spot. If the spot isn't sore, the partner moves one thumb's-width in toward the center of the skull and presses again, asking "Is that sore?"

- When a sore spot is found, the partner pushes their thumb into it for seven seconds. The partner should push hard—it should feel a little painful—but not so hard as to be excruciating. It's up to the patient to tell the partner if they are pushing too hard, and for the partner to back off if they are.

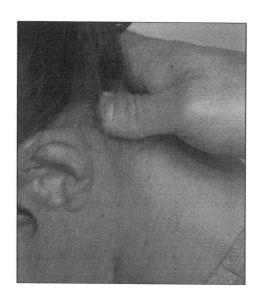

- The partner should work from left to right, working all along the base of the skull.

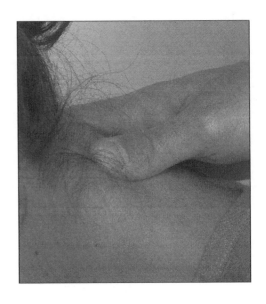

- When the partner gets to the center of the skull, they should continue to support the patient's head while the patient takes three deep breaths in and out through their nose and out through their mouth. Each time they let a breath out the patient should let their head drop forward and let their neck and shoulder muscles completely relax.

- Now it's time to work down the sides of the neck. The partner will begin looking for trigger points at a point just beneath the skull, and about an inch out from the center of the spine (find the center of the spine by using your fingertips to find the hard "bumps" in the center of the neck). The partner works from the skull to the base of the neck. The thumb should be pressed down into any trigger points that are found, again for seven seconds.

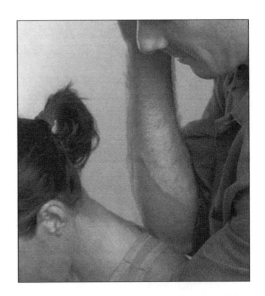

- Once the neck is complete, it's time to work on the shoulders. The partner can continue to use their thumb, but it's often easier to switch to their elbows, using the elbow to find the trigger points, and using the weight of their body to put pressure into the points.

- Once done with the left side, the partner should repeat the work on his patient's right side.

- Note: Trigger points usually don't move, and you'll usually have three to six of them most involved with your headaches and neck pain. After awhile, the partner may get to know the patient's neck well enough to go right to those trigger points most involved with triggering their neck pain and headaches.

Self Massage

Wouldn't it be nice to have a good massage at your fingertips? You do! Here's the best way to rub the kinks out of your own neck and shoulders:

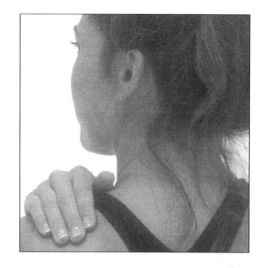

- Cup your right hand and move it to the left shoulder. Starting at the base of your neck, begin squeezing the top of your shoulder. Work your way out toward the end of the shoulder, squeezing each section 2-3 times. Now work your way back up toward the neck.

- When you have finished, flatten your hand and press your fingers together so that you can use the tips of your fingers to dig deep into your shoulder muscles. Start at the base of the neck and, using a circular motion, dig the tips of your fingers into the tops and backs of your shoulder muscles. Keep digging as you move out to the end of your shoulder, concentrating on any tight spots.

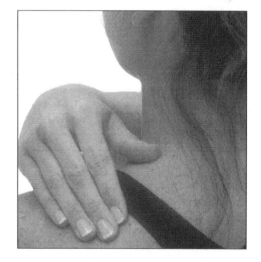

- Now find the tightest spot and, using the tips of your fingers, dig into it. With your fingers still dug into the tight muscle, drag that area of your shoulder forward toward your chest, releasing it when your fingers slide over the top of your shoulder.

- Repeat on the left shoulder.

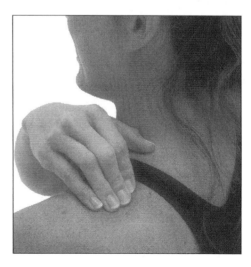

49

Resistance Stretching

Resistance stretching takes advantage of the fact that when you use your muscles they become fatigued...and easier to stretch. What you'll do is push your head against resistance in order to fatigue your neck muscles...then stretch these same muscles in the opposite direction:

- Start by sitting up straight.

- Place your right hand on the left side of your head.

- Now push your head toward your left shoulder while you resist with your right hand. You'll hold this isometric contraction for 10 seconds, all the time pushing your head toward your left shoulder while preventing your head from moving.

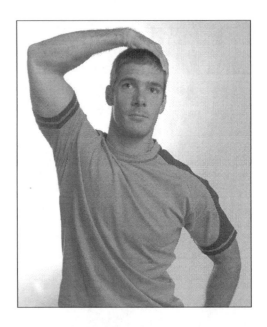

- After 10 seconds, relax, stop pushing and take a deep breath in and out. Now use your right hand and arm to gently pull your neck toward your right shoulder. USE CAUTION. Let the weight of your arm do the stretching, and only stretch as far as is comfortable. It's easy to over-do this stretch. Take three breaths in and out. Each time you let a breath out, allow your neck to stretch a little farther to the right.

- Repeat to the opposite side.

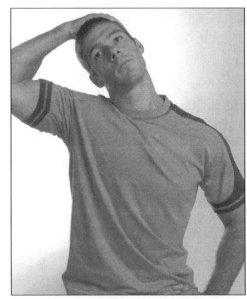

Using Tennis Balls For Neck Pain

Using tennis balls to release chronic muscular tension is one of the simplest, yet most powerful, self-help techniques ever developed. By applying pressure to specific points on your body, the surrounding muscles relax. Besides easing pain, this helps better your alignment. Best of all, the technique is fast. In only minutes you can feel a dramatic difference in the way your body feels and moves.

Headache/Top of The Neck Pain And Tension

- Begin by lying on the floor, your knees bent, feet flat on the floor. Place a tennis ball in the palm of one of your hands. Place your hand with the tennis ball in it under your head, so that the ball rests in the center of your neck, right beneath your skull (there should be a slight hollow there where the ball fits comfortably—see illustration on next page).

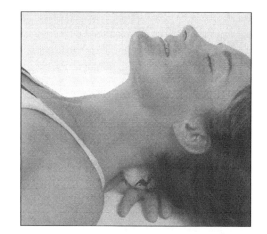

- Let your head and neck sink down into the tennis ball. This may produce an achy feeling. Rest on the ball, letting your head sink down toward the floor with every breath that you let out. After 10-30 seconds you should start to notice the achy feeling start to go away. When it does you are done with this point.

- Now take another tennis ball and put both balls in the palms of your interlocked hands so that the balls touch. Again, rest your head on the balls so they are centered and right beneath your skull. Your head should feel like it is "falling back" over the balls as they form a fulcrum at the point where your neck and head join (see illustration).

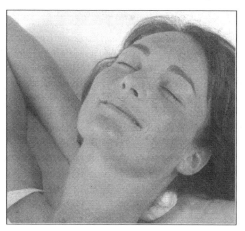

- Again, rest on the balls, letting your head sink down toward the floor with every breath you let out. After 10-30 seconds you should start to notice the achy feeling start to go away. When it does you are done with these points.

Note: If the achy feeling produced by lying on the balls becomes <u>more</u> painful as you do one of these areas, stop and try that area again some other time. Also, if the pain doesn't lessen after 30 seconds, stop and come back to the exercise at a later time.

Using Tennis Balls For Lower Neck Pain

- Now take two tennis balls and place them on either side of your spine, just below your neck, at the tops of your shoulder blades (see illustration bellow). If you can't reach far enough to place the balls in the correct spot, place them at the base of your neck and use your legs to push your body up a few inches, which will make the balls slide a few inches down your back.

- Once the balls are in place bring your hands to the opposite shoulders, giving yourself a "hug".

- Take long, slow, deep breaths as you let yourself sink down into the balls for 10-30 seconds.

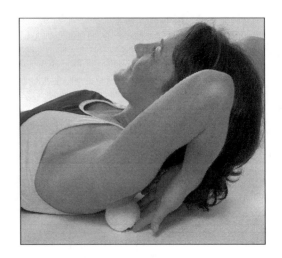

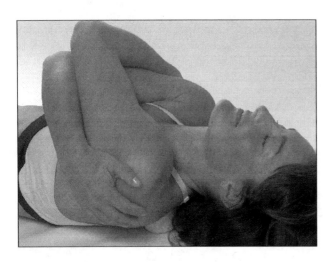

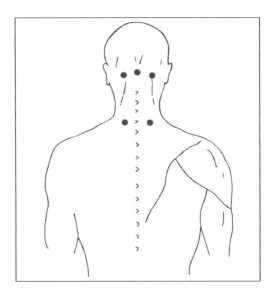

The Perfect Posture Program
Approximate Workout Time: 10 Minutes

*If you want to correct your posture, you need to work the muscles on the **back** of your body, because those are the ones that keep us upright. The Perfect Posture Program will get you standing tall and healthy again. If you have growing children the exercises will let you stop complaining about slumping shoulders and drooping stances and let you start training your children to stand in the healthiest way possible.*

The Ball Bearing

This exercise reverses the forward-bending posture by bending your body backward over a large exercise ball, available in sporting goods stores or in the exercise section of mass merchants like Wal-Mart. You may hear "pops and clicks" in your spine as you do this exercise. This is a good sign, indicating your spine is adjusting itself to a new, healthier posture. You may also notice an increase in the amount of air you can inhale.

Breathing correctly is extremely important when doing this exercise. Breathe slowly through your nose, and concentrate on how your breath flows in and out of your body. As you breathe out through your mouth, feel your muscles become more and more relaxed.

▪ Squat and position your ball so that when you lie back the ball rests between your shoulder blades.

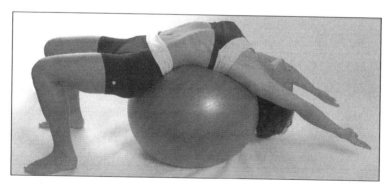

▪ Take a breath; as you slowly breathe out lie back on the ball. Let yourself relax and feel your body sink down toward the floor. Imagine that you are at the beach, that your body is made of wax, and that you're melting over a warm beach ball on the sand. Every time you breathe out, feel yourself get softer and more and more relaxed, letting yourself sink down toward the floor.

▪ Take ten slow, deep breaths. This short routine goes a long way toward reinvigorating your posture and energy level.

The Back Loop

This exercise is an antidote to civilization. Living in the modern world, most of our daily activities bend us forward. The most devastating habit is sitting, because virtually everyone sits in a way that bends them forward.

The Back Loop reverses forward bending. The key to its effectiveness is that it utilizes the back's erector muscles, which become stretched and weak in most members of our slumping society.

- Lie face down on the floor, with your hands resting close to your shoulders. Raise yourself up slightly so you can comfortably touch your chin to the floor.

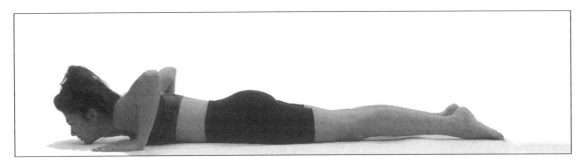

- Take a deep breath in through your nose, and as you slowly blow it out through your mouth raise your torso up off the floor while looking straight ahead. Try not to push up with your arms; use your back muscles as much as possible.

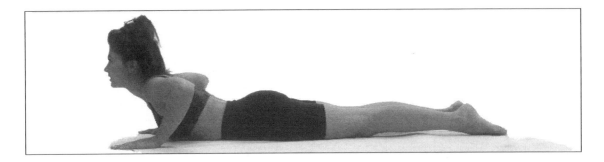

- Come up only as high as is comfortable. Because we use these muscles so little, it's best to take it easy. As your back muscles get stronger you'll be able to lift higher off the ground.

- Do five repetitions. On your fifth attempt hold your highest position and slowly breathe in and out through your nose. The first time you attempt this won't be easy; you may only be able to hold the position for a few seconds. Be gentle with yourself, and increase the last part of the exercise until you can hold the position and slowly breathe in and out three times.

The Wall Slide

Tired of slouching? The Wall Slide is designed to counteract our slumping postures. It's easy to do, and all you need is a wall (or door) to lean against.

The "slide" stretches the curves in the low back, mid back and neck, refreshing the muscles along the spine while aligning your ears, shoulders, hips and ankles:

- Stand with your feet shoulder-width apart, about six inches out from a wall (you can also use a door). Lean back against the wall.

- As you take a deep breath in, bend your knees and slide down the wall until your knees are comfortably bent.

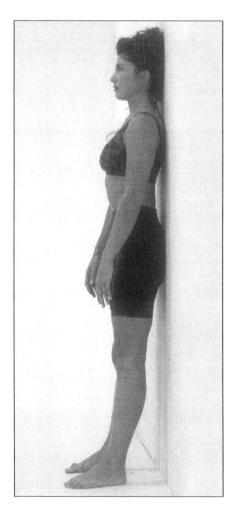

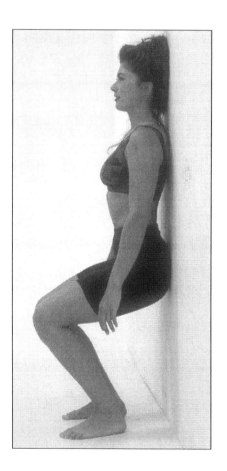

Now, press the lower part of your back, your mid-back between your shoulders, and the back of your neck against the wall.

■ After you are flat against the wall, blow your breath out slowly while sliding up the wall. (Note: You may not be able to get completely flat against the wall; try your best, but don't strain.)

Do the Wall Side four times. This is also an excellent exercise to do throughout the day to refresh your spine and posture. When finished, keep your erect posture and step away from the wall, maintaining this stance for as long as is comfortable. .

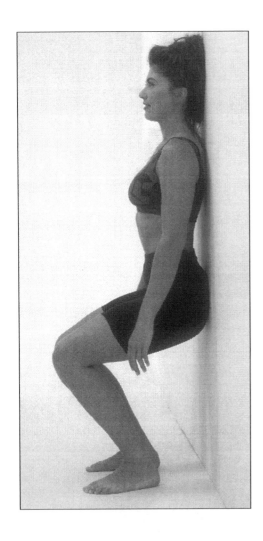 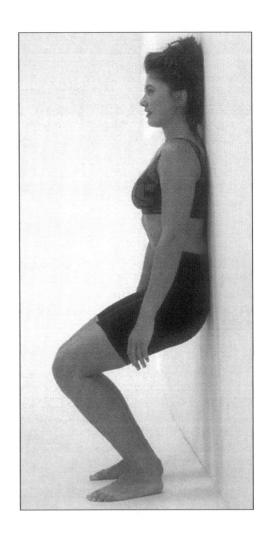

The Turtle

Few people realize how important their necks are to their well-being. Connecting your head to your body, the neck contains more nerves per square inch than any other body part.

As we have seen, if the neck is bent forward, the muscles at the back of the neck become strained trying to keep the head over the shoulders. The Turtle helps restore and keep the neck's natural curve, decreasing stress on the muscles at the back of the neck.

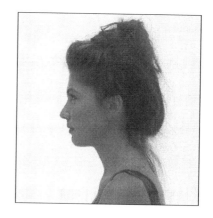

- Sit up straight in a chair or car seat. Level your chin and eyes with the horizon--you should not be looking up or down, but straight ahead.

- As you exhale, bring your chin/jaw back, keeping them parallel to the floor and hold for a count of three.

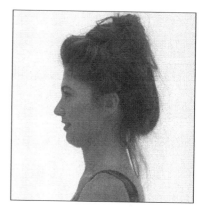

Caution: This exercise will create sore muscles if done too strenuously. Do the exercise slowly, and STOP if you experience pain. Also, the natural tendency is to tuck the chin. Don't tuck! <u>Retract</u> the neck back over the shoulders as you breathe out. Do this 10 times.

At the end of the Turtle exercise take a deep breath in; as you exhale give a long sigh, letting your chin drop to your chest. Feel the muscles at the back of your neck get a good stretch.

Note: You can help train your neck back into proper position by rolling up a small towel until it's about five inches in diameter. Wrap the roll you've made with several thick rubber bands to hold the roll's shape. Now, rest on the floor (or bed), your knees bent, the roll under your neck, for 15 minutes each day.

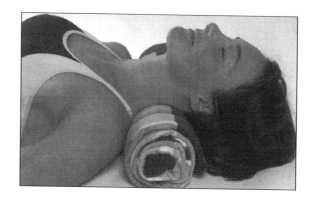

Tips for Getting and Keeping Good Posture

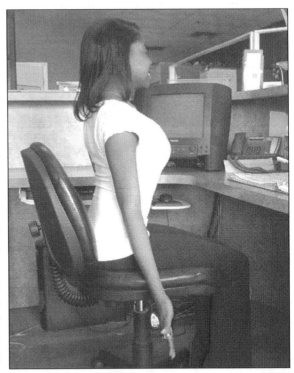

- Good posture is a must if you want optimal health, dramatically affecting your energy level and comfort. Poor posture starts as a habit; good posture is a habit, too. In the beginning you may feel strange standing and sitting in good posture. Keep at it: Good posture will become a natural habit to you.

- When working at a computer, place your monitor and papers a little below eye level; keep your eyes 18-24 inches from the monitor and rest them periodically; every 15 minutes or so look up from your work and focus on something far away— across the room or out the window.

- If working at the computer for more than an hour, do the following stretch: Sit up straight, retract your chin toward your throat, keeping your jaw parallel to the floor (don't tuck your chin). Let your arms down to your sides and straighten them. With your palms open, turn your thumbs out to the sides, at the same time contracting the muscles between your shoulder blades. Hold this position for 15 seconds (see photo above). This stretch counteracts the bad affects of sitting at a computer with your head forward and your shoulders slumped.

- Tilting your head forward just three inches in front of your shoulders triples the strain on your neck. So keep your chin level with the ground, and pull your head back so that you feel your head over your shoulders. And don't make a habit of tilting your head to one side or the other…this can cause muscle imbalances.

- When sitting, use a lumbar support (a curved, foam-filled support sold in most pharmacy departments), which will help support the curve of your low back. Place it between your back and your chair. (To make your own lumbar support: Roll a towel so that it's about 4"-5" in diameter, and then secure the towel with rubber bands to hold its shape. Slip this rolled towel between your back and your chair at your belt-line.) When reading at home you can put pillows on your chair's armrests and hold what you're reading in front of you so you don't slouch.

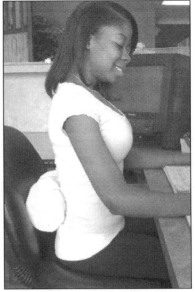

- When walking to and from your car, outside for exercise or inside on a treadmill you have a wonderful opportunity to better your posture. So walk right! Here's how: Retract your head over your shoulders and gently tense your abdominal muscles. Squeeze your shoulder blades together. As you walk, pretend there's a hot air balloon pulling your head straight toward the sky.

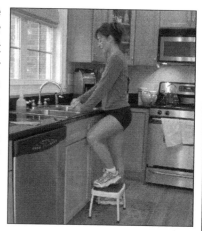

- Do this quick "posture check" throughout the day to help maintain your postural progress: Start by noticing if your ears feel like they are resting above your shoulders, rather than forward of them. Next, focus attention on your shoulders themselves. Take a deep breath, and as you exhale let your shoulders drop down toward the floor. Check your pelvis and hips, and make sure you aren't holding them so that your low back is arched backwards or tucked underneath you. Now feel that your knees aren't locked, but are freely moveable. Lastly, see that your feet are pointing forward, and that you are keeping your weight balanced on the balls of your feet.

- When standing and working, such as when washing dishes, put one foot up on a small stool or shoe box. This takes tension off your low back. If possible, raise or lower the surface on which you're working so that you can keep your neck and shoulders relaxed.

- The "Back Builder" exercise (pictured below) is possibly the single most beneficial exercise if you want to keep good posture. The reason: in order to do the exercise you need to use the muscles *on the back* of your body. These "erector spinae" muscles are the ones responsible for keeping you erect. (See a detailed description of how to do this exercise in Chapter Five.)

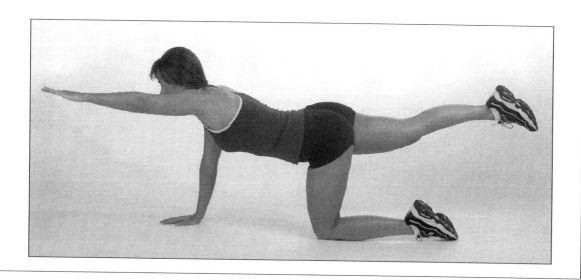

Make Your Mother Happy:
Exercising Your Way To Better Posture

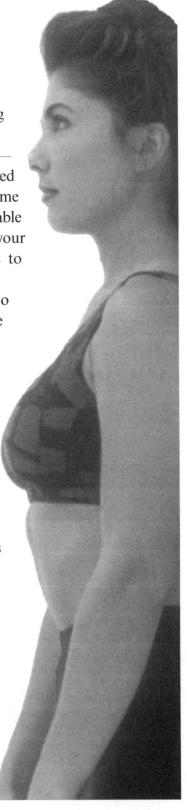

When your Mother tells you to "Stand up straight!" you hold your head up and push your shoulders back. And you stay in this upright posture--until you start to think of something else. Then your body will go right back to where it was before.

It's difficult to "think" your way to good posture. Posture—like thousands of other processes in your body, is controlled unconsciously by your nervous system. That's why the best time to concentrate on good posture is when exercising. You'll be able to keep thinking about it because you'll already be tuned into your body, and you'll have fewer distractions. But what muscles to exercise?

Your spine keeps you standing straight, but it couldn't do its job without your "antigravity muscles". These muscles are at the front and back of your body. In terms of posture, some of the most important are the erector spinae (erect spine) group, thick muscles on both sides of your spine running from your hips to the back of your head. They tend to pull you backward.

The muscles on the back of your body are so important because most of your body's weight is in front of your spine, giving you a tendency to fall forward—just what we don't want. (Think about it: Almost everything we do, we do in a "bent forward" posture. Sitting, working at the computer, driving, eating, reading, watching television—all these activities bend us forward. No wonder we end up slumped and round-shouldered as we age.)

The bottom line: To make your Mother happy you need to exercise the (often neglected) muscles on the back of your body. That way, even if you're not thinking about your posture, your muscles will be holding you in the correct position because they've been properly trained.

5 PELVIC POWER

[making the core of your body flexible and strong]

If we take a front-to-back picture of your low back and draw a line across the tops of your hips, your hips should be parallel, or level, with the floor. If your hips are uneven, with one hip higher than the other, your spine is resting on an uneven foundation, setting the stage for subluxations in your low back.

Misalignments of the bones in the low back can often be seen on the same front-to-back view of the spine. If we put a dot in the center of each of the bones on the film, they should be lined up nice and straight, perpendicular to the floor. When bones are subluxated, they are often twisted off the center line.

When subluxations take hold in our low backs, pain can become our constant, unwanted, companion. You've probably seen or heard the statistic: 80 percent of us will experience significant low back pain at some point in our

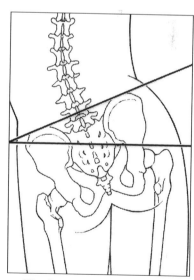

The Leaning Tower of Pisa Effect. Spinal misalignments often develop as a result of an unlevel pelvis

61

lives. It's the most common reason for lost work time and the second most common reason (behind respiratory infections) for a trip to the doctor.

Most patients want to know how their hips and low backs get out of alignment. There is no cookbook answer. Maybe their mother had a difficult time delivering them as a baby, and their skeleton has been misaligned since birth. Perhaps they fell off a bike or down some stairs. Maybe their low back became misaligned while playing sports. Maybe there is an emotional/mental or even a chemical cause to their subluxations. How your bones become misaligned isn't as important as getting them re-aligned so that nerve pressure is eliminated and your body can function the way Nature intended.

Power Center

What makes tight muscles in the back so agonizing is that they are some of the most powerful muscles in your body. Every time they contract your head, shoulders, arms and legs all respond, as if someone shook the base of a tree and all its branches shuddered. When working correctly, the low back muscles do most of the work when you get up, sit down, bend or twist. If they become tight, your body can develop problems as far away as your fingertips and toes.

Unfortunately, few of our daily activities exercise the low back muscles to keep them flexible and strong. Sitting in chairs is a good example. Studies show there are far fewer back problems in cultures where people squat on the ground rather than sit in chairs. X-ray studies of such "squatters" show their chair-less lifestyles help produce good posture and fewer back problems.

In our society our lifestyles often lead to low back muscles that are weak yet tight, increasing the chance of subluxations developing.

And let's face it: many of us create a strain on our low backs because we are overweight. As our bellies get bigger, they drag the low back forward, jamming joints in the area. (When we lose pounds or tighten our stomachs through exercise we take pressure from our low backs.)

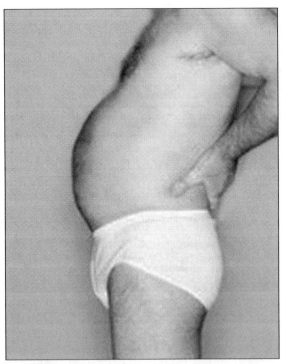

Extra weight pulls our low backs forward, jamming joints.

Your low back is a marvelous blend of strength and flexibility. Like a tree trunk it should be strong. Like bamboo it should bend. Among all the treatments for low back pain, chiropractic has been shown to be the most effective, because it focuses on improving *the function* of your low back.

The Back Pain Relief routine outlined below is designed to make your low back function better by increasing its ability to support you and allow you to move freely. It helps your back work better as a whole rather than treat specific joint, muscle, nerve or disc problems.

The Back Pain Relief Routine
Approximate workout time: 10 minutes

The Knee Pull Stretch

* Lay on your back, preferably on the floor. (You can do this exercise in bed, but your results will be less dramatic.) Raise your knees up in the air and grab them with your hands. If you've lifted your head off the ground in order to reach your knees, let your head drop back down.

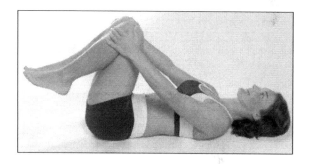

* Take a deep breath in; as you breathe out let your shoulders and neck muscles relax and pull your knees gently toward your chest. You should feel a good stretch in the muscles of your lower back. Don't strain. When you get to the point where you start to feel pain, stop and let the rest of your breath out.

* Breath in again as you let your knees drop away from your chest. Go slow! Don't force your sore back muscles to stretch beyond the point of pain. Let them relax and try to feel the tension drain out of them.

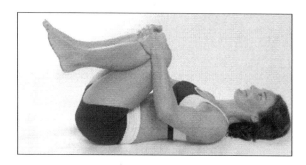

* Repeat five times.

The Deep Tilt

■ Begin by lying on the floor with your knees bent. Let your shoulders and waist relax. Take a deep breath in. As you breathe out, press the small of your back to the floor and tilt your waist up, trying to bring the tops of your hips up toward your chin. To do this you'll need to contract your stomach and buttock muscles. Move slowly and smoothly.

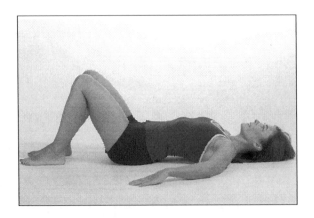

■ Inhale as you let your waist drop back down toward the floor. Let the small of your back relax.

■ Exhale and repeat the tilting motion.

■ Repeat five times.

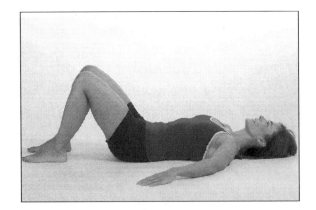

■ As your muscles get stronger and your pain fades you may want to gently lift your buttocks off the floor as you press the small of your back into the floor and tilt your pelvis up, increasing the benefit of this exercise.

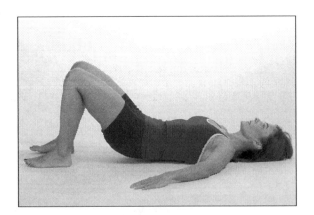

The Side to Side

- Begin by lying on the floor, your knees bent at a 45-degree angle, your arms at shoulder height, outstretched to the side (see photo on right).

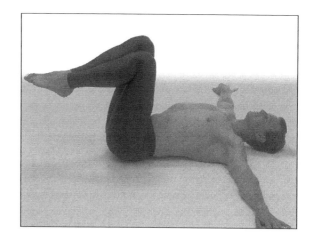

- Take a deep breath in. As you slowly exhale let your chin drop to the left while your knees drop to the right. Keep the knees together. Only drop them as far as is comfortable. Inhale as you return to the starting position. As you exhale, drop your chin to the right as your knees drop to the left. Inhale and return to the starting position. Repeat three times to each side.

- When you feel you can handle more stretch, modify the exercise: Start with your legs resting on the floor. Lift one leg up toward the ceiling, keeping it straight. Wrap a belt or rope around the ball of your foot. Hold the belt with the opposite hand, and use the belt to bring your leg over your body (see photo at right).

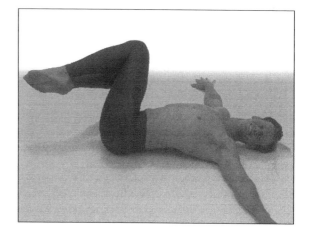

- Once your leg is fully extended and you're getting a good stretch through your hips, breath in and out slowly three times, each time letting your leg drop further toward the floor.

- Repeat to the other side.

Note: For more information, see Hip Stretch With A Belt in the "Help For Your Hips" section of this book.

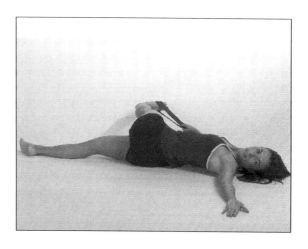

The Bicycle

This is an excellent exercise for people who have tight hamstrings--the large muscles running from the back of your knees to the bottom of your buttocks. Tight hamstrings are common in people who sit at a desk most of the day and often contribute to low back pain.

■ Begin by lying on your back. Raise your knees up to your chest and grab the sides of your feet, wrapping your hands around the outside of them. You may have to stretch and raise your head off the floor to get a grip on your feet. Once you do, relax and let your head drop back to the floor.

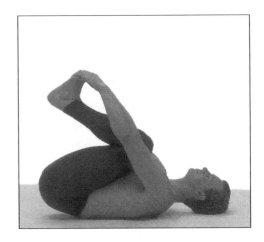

■ Start with the left leg and push it out, attempting to straighten the leg. Stop when the leg won't extend further. Count "One". As you bring the left leg back toward your chest push the right leg out, again stretching to its limit. Count "Two".

■ Repeat the bicycle motion to a count of 50, pushing out with one leg, then the other. Keep your head on the floor and don't strain. It may take several weeks for you to fully extend your legs during this exercise.

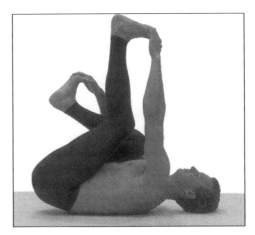

Note: If you can't reach your toes to do this exercise, do The Hamstring Stretch exercise described in the "Help For Your Knees" section of this book. Also, see the first section of the Hip Stretch With A Belt exercise in the a"Help For Your Hips" section. Using a belt, anyone can get a good hamstring stretch.

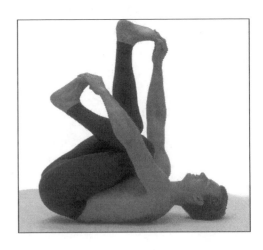

The Back Builder

We live in a society in which we are constantly bending forward. The only way to strengthen our back muscles, however, is to use them to bend us backward. The Back Builder does just that. However, don't attempt this exercise until you are almost completely out of pain. If you try it and it causes pain, stop and wait a week or two before trying it again.

- Start on all fours, with your body in the shape of a table--arms and thighs straight down, perpendicular to the floor. You should be looking straight ahead. Find a spot on the wall or, if outside, on a distant fixed spot.

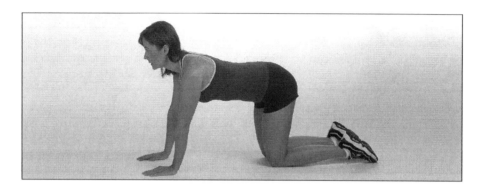

- Taking a breath in, extend your left arm out and your right leg back, "dragging" them along the floor. As you breathe out, raise your arm to shoulder level and your leg to waist level. Hold them in this position as you take in and let out two breaths. Inhale as you bring the arm and leg down to the floor; exhale as you resume the starting pose.

- Taking a breath in, repeat the exercise with your right arm out and your left leg back.

- Repeat three times to each side. As you progress, increase the time you hold the position. Build to the point where you can hold your arms and legs up for eight full breaths.

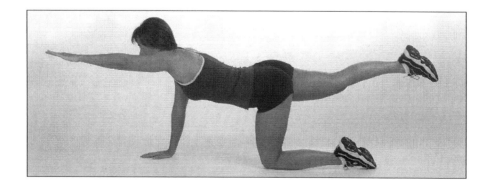

Using Tennis Balls for Back Pain/Sciatica

Tennis balls are a great tool to relieve tight muscles in your back and buttocks.

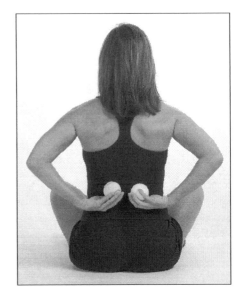

- Lie on your back with your feet flat on the floor. Take two tennis balls and place them on either side of your spine, just below your ribcage (see photo at right for the correct placement). The balls should press into the muscles on either side of your spine.

- Fold your arms in front of your body, opening up the shoulder blades and ribcage. Take deep, slow breaths. Each time you breathe out let your body sink down into the balls. Continue to let yourself sink down into the balls for one minute. Stop if the balls become uncomfortable.

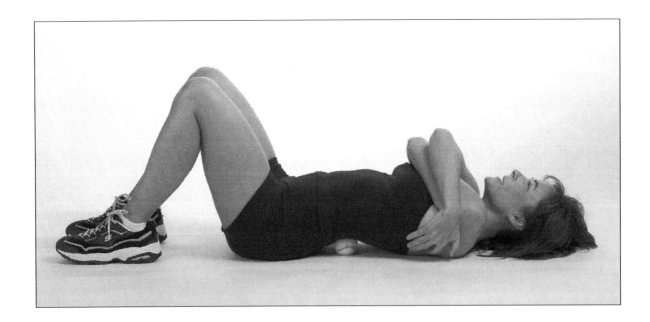

Now, lie on your back with your feet flat on the floor. Take two tennis balls and place them under your back, on either side of your spine, right at the belt line. The balls should press up into your tight back muscles.

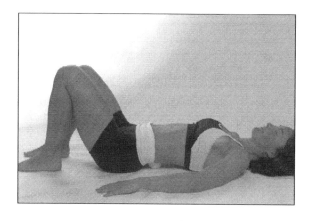

Using your feet to maneuver, gently rock your body from side to side, so that the tennis balls move across your low back. They should only move two or three inches, and should not roll over your spine.

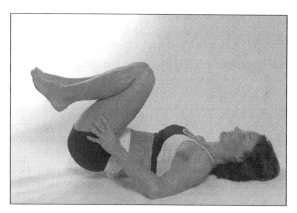

To have the balls push more deeply into your back, bring your legs up toward your chest (see photo at right). This also allows you to more easily move your body over the balls by using your hands to push your thighs from side to side.

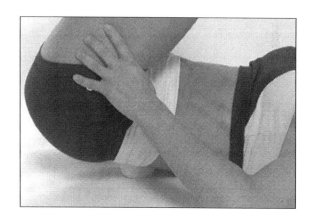

Continue gently rolling the balls over your low back for one to two minutes. Stop if doing this exercise causes undo pain, but you should feel the balls digging into the muscles (most people say it's a "good" pain).

▪ Next, take the tennis balls away and lay on your back. Starting with the left leg, place a single tennis ball in the upper third of your buttock (see photo at right).

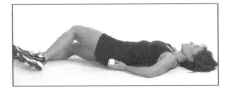

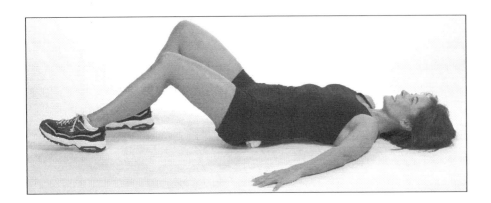

▪ Straighten your left leg and lower it to the floor as you lay flat on your back. Keep your right leg bent. Using your bent leg for leverage, roll slightly to the left so that the tennis ball "digs into" your buttock. Move over the tennis ball, finding the area that is most tight and painful. Gently roll the ball into the tightest spot, using your legs to vary the pressure on the ball. This can be quite painful; continue rolling on the ball to your tolerance level for one minute.

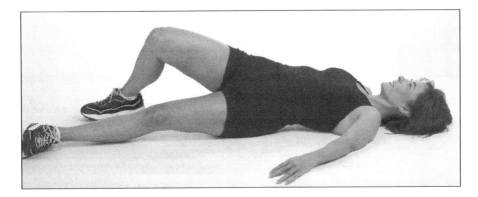

▪ Switch sides and do the right buttock.

Note: This is a particularly effective exercise for pain that starts in the low back and travels down the leg. If one leg hurts more than the other, do that leg first.

Stomach Crunches

Think of your stomach as the front of your back. Since your low back is curved forward, extra weight on the front of your body exaggerates the spine's natural curve, jamming joints at the rear of the spine. Strong abdominal muscles help keep this from happening. This exercise gets its name from the way you'll be crunching together your abdominals:

- Start by lying on the floor, your knees bent, feet flat on the floor. Clasp your hands together at the back of your head. Relax your shoulders.

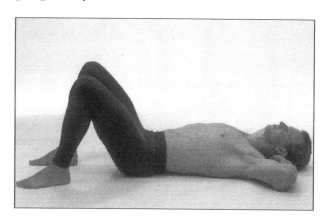

- Take a breath, and as you exhale raise your torso up off the floor far enough so that your shoulder blades just lift off the floor. (You might find it easier to do crunches if you imagine a large red arrow suspended above your belly, pointing straight down toward your belly button. As you breathe out, imagine the arrow pressing into your abdomen and let this imaginary force raise you up.)

- Exhale and resume the starting position.

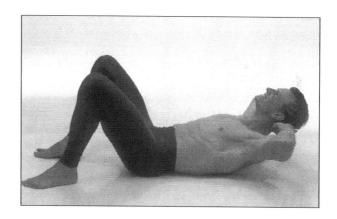

- Keep your arms relaxed, with your elbows dropped down toward the floor. It's natural to want to pull your elbows up toward your knees. Avoid this; let them stay out to the sides.

- Start with five stomach crunches and work your way up to 25 each day. And remember, as with most exercises, the number of repititions isn't as important as doing the exercise correctly: Better form produces better results.

Note: It's important not to tuck your chin or strain your neck as you do your crunches. To keep your head and neck in the proper position, imagine an apple tucked under your chin and don't let your chin crush this apple as you raise yourself off the floor.

Sitting Back Stretch

This is an excellent stretch to do anytime you're sitting and your back feels tight:

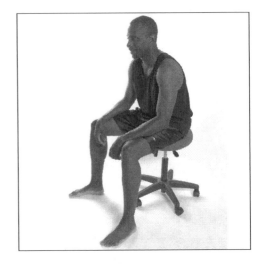

- Sit up straight at the edge of a chair. Place your elbows on your knees. Turn your right hand in so that your thumb is pointing to the right and your palm is facing out; let your arm drop so that the web of your right hand rests on top of your right ankle (see photo on right).

- Supporting yourself with your right arm, let your left hand drop to your left ankle. Again, turn your hand as shown. Using your arms for support, take a deep breath in, and as you slowly blow the air out let your torso drop between your legs. You should feel a good stretch in your low back.

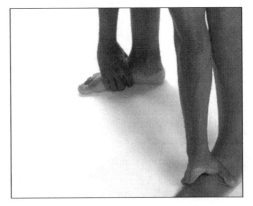

- Once you are in the position described above, try this: As you breathe in, stretch your torso up and out, stretching your head and torso as far out from your lower back as possible. As you breathe out, let your head, neck and torso drop down toward the floor, feeling the stretch in your lower back.

- Start with three long, slow, deep, breaths, letting your head and torso sink further toward the floor with every breath you let out. Eventually increase the number of breaths, building up to as many as are comfortable.

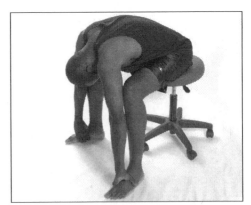

How to Lift

Most lifting injuries occur because we don't think before we hoist a heavy load. Before beginning a lift, plan on accomplishing five actions:

▪ Bend your knees and lift with your legs. Transferring stress from your back to the large muscles of your legs is the best way to prevent injury.

▪ Tighten your abdominal muscles. Tightening the "abs" transfers tension from your low back to your belly, forming a "girdle" of muscle around your waist that protects your back.

▪ Get close to the object you're lifting. This helps your balance. Keeping the weight close to your center of gravity also transfers stress from your arms and back to your legs.

▪ Avoid twisting while lifting. If you need to move an object to the right or left, keep your torso over your hips and feet and take several "baby steps" in the direction you need to go.

▪ Keep your shoulders back. This will help keep your back straight, allowing your spine to maintain its natural, strength-giving curves.

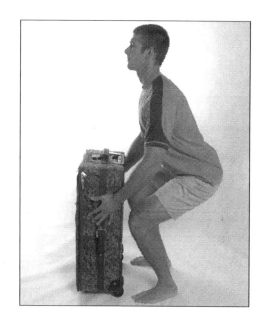

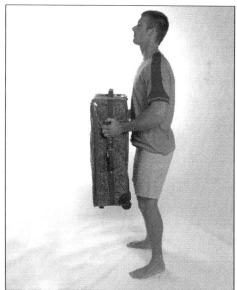

Back Brace Talk

Do back braces work? Are they right for you?

Yes, back braces do work to stabilize your low back. They are particularly helpful when your back pain is worse upon movement. This is the sort of pain that comes from a sprain or strain of the back muscles. By stabilizing the area with a brace these injured muscles don't have to work so hard and they have an easier time relaxing.

There are two schools of thought concerning wearing back braces on the job, even if you don't have pain. One says you shouldn't wear them on a consistent basis because doing so will allow your back muscles to soften and become more prone to injury. The other says that by supporting your back you prevent yourself from making ill-advised moves and injuring yourself. Both are valid viewpoints, and it depends on the patient's particular condition as to whether they will benefit from a back brace or sacroiliac belt.

6 HIGH VOLTAGE

[boosting your power supply with proper nutrition]

Food For Thought

There is a magical intelligence inside of you. It's striving 24 hours a day to keep you healthy by turning the food you eat into all the chemicals and energy you need to stay healthy. It can take peanut butter sandwiches and cucumbers and turn them into muscles and heart tissue. The more help you give this incredible force inside of you, the quicker you'll experience abundant health. It's a fact: By eating well your nervous system will function better, your spine will get in alignment faster and you will be in less pain.

In this chapter you'll learn how and what to eat in order to get and stay healthy, including:

- How your digestive system works
- Basic rules for eating
- What food and "pretend foods" you must avoid or limit in order to stay healthy
- How and when to use proteins, carbohydrates and fats
- How to handle digestive problems
- Vitamins and herbs your body and nervous system crave
- Using natural supplements to heal common health complaints
- Eating to get out of pain
- Eating and breathing for energy
- Eating and breathing to relax

Fast Track

How does a banana get turned into energy your body can use to thrive? Food starts being transformed into energy when you chew. As your teeth grind and mash, saliva lubricates what you're eating and starts breaking down starches (for example, pasta and potatoes).

Once swallowed your meal slides into your stomach. There it's squeezed and mixed with chemicals to break it down further. Some of the most important chemicals are **digestive enzymes** (used to "unlock" chemical bonds so food falls apart). Many raw foods contain the enzymes your body needs to break them down. Without the proper enzymes, your body has a tough time…food can stay undigested, leading to problems.

Different foods pass through the stomach at different rates. For example, carbohydrates like fruits, vegetables and breads are digested quickly. Proteins like meat and beans take longer. Fatty foods like the skin on fried chicken take the longest of all. Cold foods slow the stomach down while hot foods speed it up. Drinks, on the other hand, usually flow through the stomach. (So to get something into your system quickly, dissolve it in warm liquid).

Once your stomach turns what you've eaten into a liquid, it pushes it into your small intestine, which is about 22 feet long in adults and thicker than a rubber inner tube. As food enters the intestine more breakdown chemicals are added to it and digestion really gets going, with food that once ranged from chocolate covered ants to charcoal broiled zucchini getting broken into a handful of basic chemicals. These chemicals are then transported through the intestinal walls into your bloodstream.

After a journey of 12 to 48 hours or more through the stomach and small intestine, unabsorbed "food" travels into the colon, where water and salt are removed and over a dozen different strains of friendly bacteria break down what's left. The excess is then eliminated.

Note: The following advice will develop good eating habits that will allow most people to thrive. However, if you suffer from low blood sugar, diabetes or other diseases, or if you want to lose or gain weight, you'll need to talk with a health professional qualified in nutritional matters before making any dietary changes.

[Eating Etiquette]

Think of food as a beautifully wrapped gift. Inside is a wonderful present. It's gold and shining and gives off a warm glow. The energy in wholesome food is like that. To get it out, we need a digestive system functioning like a 5-year-old on Christmas morning, ripping off wrappings to get to the good stuff inside.

Because a healthy digestive tract is crucial if you want to wring maximum energy from your food, you need to treat it right. Following are some guidelines for keeping your digestive system in top shape.

Eat Natural

Recently I had a very nice woman in her late-40's come to me as a new patient. She was on eight prescription medications for several chronic pain syndromes. She was under the care of four different specialists for her health problems. I asked her to write a "diet diary" to see if what she was or wasn't eating might be contributing to her health problems. She began on Monday morning. Her first entry read "Breakfast: Pop Tarts".

If what I'm about to say to you comes as a surprise then I'm glad you're finally hearing it from me: If you have a lot of health problems, you are going to have a very hard time getting well eating Pop Tarts for breakfast.

With all the nutrition information available today, the most important information about diet and nutrition is sometimes lost: If you eat natural foods--meaning they actually grow in nature--they will contain everything your body needs to break the food down, take the nutrients your body needs, and eliminate what your body doesn't need in the most efficient way possible. This will save your body energy it can use for healing and thriving.

On the other hand, if you eat breakfast or dinner from a box, your body has to struggle mightily to get any nutrition from these "meals". When you eat artificial food, not only doesn't it give you nutrition you can use for healing, it drags you down. It chugs through your body as "dead weight," robbing you of energy as your body tries desperately to find something in it of value.

So, the number one rule of eating right is this: Eat as much food as you possibly can in its natural state. The farther from its natural state, the less the food will help you to thrive.

Natural Foods Are Best!

Apples, bananas, blackberries, blueberries, cantaloupe, grapefruit, grapes, kiwis, nectarines, oranges, peaches, pears, pineapple, plums, prunes, raisins, raspberries, strawberries, watermelon, whole-grain breads, brown rice, oatmeal, rice cakes, corn, peas, potatoes, squash, alfalfa sprouts, artichokes, asparagus, avocados, beets, broccoli, cabbage, carrots, celery, cucumbers, eggplant, green beans, lettuce, olives, radishes, spinach, string beans, tomatoes, zucchini, beans, almonds, walnuts, flax, sesame, and sunflower seeds, eggs, fish, chicken, lean beef…get the idea?

Drink Water

Your body is 70% water, so it makes sense that most of the food you eat should be water-rich. This is one reason why fruits and vegetables are so good for us: most contain lots of water.

Only about 30% of what you eat should be concentrated, low-water content foods like meat, bread, grains, dairy products and starches. While these foods provide essential nutrients, eating too much of them saps energy because they are much harder for you to digest.

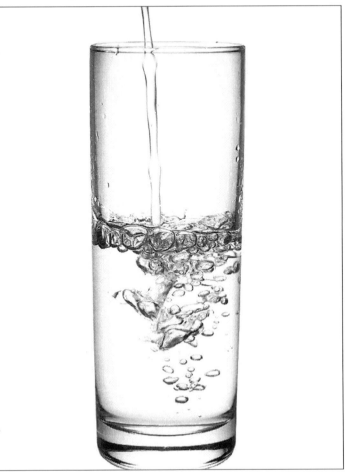

Another word on water: If you want your body to heal, you must water it. If you did nothing more than drink eight glasses of water each day, within a week you would probably notice a positive change in your health. We are a nation of chronically dehydrated people. Even if you don't want to make drinking eight glasses of water each day a habit for life, you owe it to yourself to make it a daily routine for one month to jump-start your personal healing process.

Eat Less

Stuffing yourself strains your system's ability to digest what you eat. Also, overeating drains energy. You may have noticed that after a large lunch or dinner nothing is more appealing than a long nap. That's because in order to digest large meals your body diverts blood to the stomach and intestines from other areas of your body, including your brain. The more food you eat, the less alert you are.

Eat In A Peaceful Atmosphere

As Deepak Chopra writes in his bestselling book, "Perfect Health": "Your body is tremendously alert while you are eating. Your stomach cells are aware of the conversation at the dinner table, and if they hear harsh words, the stomach will know the distress."

Eat In A Comfortable Position

Consuming food while you're standing, walking or driving can lead to indigestion because your body can't concentrate on breaking down the food you've eaten.

Eat Only When You're Hungry

Sure, eating chocolate might feel good when you're tense, but that's a sure way to put on pounds and produce burps and gas.

Avoid Ice Cold And Piping Hot Food And Drink

These will alter your stomach's normal actions.

Chew Your Food Slowly And Thoroughly

Digestion starts in the mouth, so get it off to a good start by turning your food to mush before you swallow.

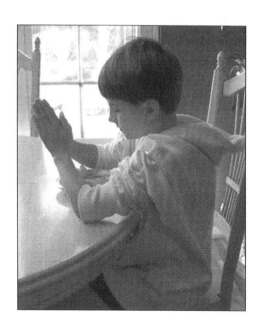

Limit How Much You Drink With Your Food

Drinking a lot of water or other beverages with your food dilutes the juices your stomach produces to digest your food.

Bless Your Food

Studies show that an "attitude of gratitude" when it comes to the food we eat helps us digest it better.

Killing You Harshly

There isn't space enough in this book to list all the "Pop Tart-like" products out there lining supermarket shelves and killing us with their empty promises as they masquerade as food. Some special villains need exposing, however. These "foods" are everywhere, and create an enormous strain on any body unlucky enough to ingest them. Here are the worst offenders:

Sugar And Sugar Substitutes

While you may love the taste of sugar, your body just can't handle it well. The makers of sugar take sugarcane and process it. And process it. And process it. By the time it gets into the candy bars, packaged foods and drinks that fill up so many stomachs every day it's completely devoid of nutritional value.

Refined sugar has been linked to all kinds of health problems, including abnormal brain function, depression, and diabetes, just to name a few. Of course, sugar contains a lot of calories, too, and your body has an easy time turning sugar to fat. So it's also at the root of many people's weight problems.

Because we all know, even if we don't like to admit it, that sugar is bad for us, many of us think, "Since sugar is so bad, I'll use sugar substitutes like Sweet 'N Low." Don't do it! Sugar substitutes are even worse than the real thing! Entire books have been written linking these pretend sweeteners to health problems ranging from allergies to decreased brain function. Sugar substitutes are manufactured in huge vats in huge factories. When you ingest them, your body has to work really hard to detoxify itself.

So, how can you have your sweets and your health, too? Use honey and maple syrup when you want to sweeten your drinks or food. Avoid white sugar and artificial sweeteners just as you would pesticides, because your body reacts to them in much the same way.

Artificial Food Additives and Preservatives

Oh, the wonders of modern science! Let's take something like wheat, growing like it was going out of style in a field that is a golden example of Nature's handiwork. Let's harvest the wheat, grind it, mash it, cook it, and mix it with sixteen different chemicals the boys down at the lab came up with so it can sit on a shelf for a near eternity. Then lets spray a mixture of sugar and three other chemicals on it, put it in a box, and give it to our kids for breakfast!

Again, chemicals from "the boys in the lab" do your body absolutely no good. When you eat this stuff your body tries very hard to process it, but guess what: If a chemical was made to preserve or in some way alter food, when it gets into your system this same chemical will try its hardest to have the same effect on the inside of your body! The less food additives, artificial food flavorings and fake food color you eat, the better.

Junk Food

Fast food, including virtually the whole menu at fast food restaurants (sodas, hamburgers, French fries, fried chicken) and packaged foods (cookies, chips, and other snacks from the "snack" isle of the supermarket) are full of things your body can't use and devoid of anything your body can use to get healthy. Eating a lot of fast and refined foods is about the easiest way to get fat and unhealthy, because these foods take a tremendous toll on your body. If the fat in these foods doesn't get you, the artificial ingredients will.

Likewise with "white foods" such as white rice, white pasta and baked goods (white bread and pastries) made from white flour. These foods have had all the vitamins and other nutrients processed out of them. Because they are nutritionally dead, they clog your system without giving you the nutrition you crave in return.

The worst ingredients you'll find on the snack food isle are "hydrogenated" and "partially hydrogenated" oils. These oils are used to keep baked goods and packaged foods from melting and spoiling at room temperature. In your body, however, they contribute to heart and circulatory problems. Stay away from them as much as possible by searching for items that don't contain them.

Too Many Dairy Products

Most people are somewhat aware of the dangers of sugar and processed foods. But I find many patients don't realize that they need to be cautious when it comes to milk and milk products. "But doctor, what about those ads showing celebrities with their cute milk mustaches? And Mom always told me to drink my milk. Surely milk and cheese can't be bad!"

The truth is--despite what the multi-million dollar ad campaigns from the diary producers would have you believe--too much milk and other diary products cause a lot of people a lot of health problems.

Before you dismiss this thought, think of this: Cow's milk was made for baby cows. If you look at its composition, it contains lots of very large protein molecules, which are perfect if you're trying to grow a cow, but can cause problems when you're trying to eat in the healthiest way possible. Also, milk is pasteurized, which not only kills off germs, but kills off many of the nutrients in milk that might be good for you. Studies show that baby calves raised on pasteurized milk are sickly! And if this weren't enough, most of the cows that we get our milk from are injected or fed a host of chemicals. These range from antibiotics to hormones to keep cows growing fast and to prevent diseases that could spread to other cows. These chemicals get passed into the diary products we drink and eat.

O.K., so now you might be getting the idea that drinking a glass of milk a day might not be the healthiest thing for you. But you may still be having this thought: What about my bones? Doesn't milk build strong bones and teeth? The truth is, you'd be better off getting your calcium from green leafy vegetables. The calcium from vegetables is much easier for your body to absorb, and the veggies help create an environment in your body conducive to bone growth.

What problems do diary products cause? I find them associated with many digestive and allergy ailments. In adults, many digestive complaints fade away when milk is eliminated from the diet. And the majority of children who come into my practice with allergies and chronic ear infections do dramatically better when their parents switch to soy or rice milk.

Too Much Meat

There is really only one fact you need to know about eating a lot of meat: When different populations around the world are studied to see who is healthiest, big meat-eaters never live as long as big vegetable eaters. The reason: your body has to work very hard to digest meat. While fat takes the longest to leave your stomach, protein takes more total digestion time than any other food. That's why high-protein diets let you lose weight: your body burns a lot of calories just to break down meat and other high-protein foods. Over time, however, the wear and tear on your body is tremendous.

There are other reasons why meat isn't healthy in large quantities. One is that most of the meat in supermarkets comes from huge commercial operations where cows, chickens, pigs and turkeys are raised in cramped spaces and fed hormones and other drugs to make them grow fast and disease-free. Good for business. But the meat isn't nearly the same as when animals grow up under the sun, eating from fields. Studies show that the meat from commercially raised animals contains more "bad" fat and is higher in cholesterol.

The solution, again, is to eat more fruits and vegetables. (Note: High protein diets are very popular, and they work for many people to lose weight. However, once the weight is gone most authorities recommend cutting back on meat and dairy products.) So, limit the amount of meat you eat. Eating one serving of meat about the size of the palm of your hand each day is a good rule of thumb. To get more protein, eat more beans, nuts, seeds, and soy products like tofu, and soy-based protein drinks.

Too Much Caffeine

Caffeine is a drug, and a powerful one at that. Like all drugs, it should be used cautiously. Energy and alertness can be "bought" with coffee, tea and caffeinated soft drinks, but at a high price.

For example, one reason the caffeine in coffee and soda is so effective is that it rushes into your bloodstream and blocks the action of chemicals that normally slow down your nervous system. It's as if you cut the brake lines on a car traveling down a mountain. Nerves fire more rapidly, and your body roars to life. Most people don't have a problem with coffee. In fact, drinking coffee may have some health benefits. Some coffee drinkers, however, experience an increased susceptibility to sleeplessness, restlessness, and "burned out" feelings.

While coffee itself might be harmless, putting sugar or sugar substitutes in your coffee (and perhaps dairy products or artificial dairy products), isn't healthy. And relying on caffeine for energy puts you on an "energy roller coaster" every day. In the morning you drink coffee or soda, sending nerve impulses crackling through your body. Bingo! Instant energy. But within a few hours the caffeine wears off and, feeling like someone has cut the wires to your battery, you hit the coffeepot or soda machine for another "fix". And so it goes…from energy high to energy pothole, up and down throughout the day. By eating right it's possible to get off the energy roller coaster. You still may drink a coffee or soda once in awhile, but you won't feel like you need them just to get through the day.

Cafeteria Plan

The greatest nutritionist in the world is already inside you, turning everything from sandwiches to spumoni into energy every day. This nutritional guru works with three basic types of foods to keep you healthy: carbohydrates, proteins, and fats. (Vegetables are usually thought of as carbohydrates, and this is confusing to some people because of the bad reputation carbohydrates have earned. It's sometimes easier to think of vegetables as their very own food group. Unlike other carbs-- and proteins and fats-- you can pretty much eat all the vegetables you want, day or night.)

Understanding the healthiest way to eat means knowing what kinds of foods do what for you. And knowing how and when to eat them. The very same food you eat in the morning for energy might make you fat if you eat it as a late night snack. When you get savvy about eating your carbohydrates, proteins and fats in the right way at the right time, your body starts to really hum. You're maximizing the value of your food, which in turn maximizes your energy and ability to heal.

Cracking The Carbohydrate Code

If you were a carbohydrate you might feel like an innocent man accused of a vicious crime. Everybody tries to blame his or her fat on you. In truth, carbohydrates are good guys. They are your body's most efficient source of energy. Many people run into trouble with carbs because your body easily breaks them down into sugar. If you don't burn the sugar, your body stores it as fat. Also, if you have excess fat and continue to eat carbs, your body can lose the ability to regulate the sugar in your blood, and you can develop diabetes. So handling carbs correctly is one of the most important skills in eating well.

The main types of carbohydrates are fruits (apples, bananas, grapefruit, peaches, etc.), vegetables (broccoli, carrots, celery, green beans, potatoes, etc.), and grains (whole wheat bread, whole grain cereals, brown rice, oatmeal, etc.).

How should you eat carbs? As with all other foods, the fresher, the better. For example, old-fashioned oatmeal that takes five minutes to cook is better than the stuff that comes in a microwavable packet. Fresh fruits are better than canned. Steamed or lightly sautéed broccoli is better than a broccoli casserole that's been baked for 45 minutes.

When should you eat carbs? By far the best time to eat fruit is in the morning. It's light, so it won't slow you down. It gives quick energy. And when you eat it in the morning, you have all day to burn off the sugar from fruit. Also, fruit doesn't digest well when mixed with protein and/or fat, so it's best to eat fruit by itself.

Some people with sugar problems don't do well with fruit in the morning. They are better off having a complex carbohydrate like oatmeal or whole-wheat toast, which break down less quickly, keeping their blood sugar more stable. Grains are good for breakfast, lunch or dinner, depending on what else you're eating.

Vegetables, on the other hand, can be eaten any time. They don't present the same sugar problems as fruit, and combine well with other foods. Spinach for breakfast? Go for it!

Protein Power

Much of your body is made of proteins. As you go through your day certain body tissues are damaged. When you eat proteins they are broken into amino acids, which your body then uses to rebuild itself. Simply put, you need proteins to repair your body.

Fish, chicken, beans, soy products, protein drinks, beef, eggs and diary products are loved by people looking to lose weight fast. Why? Because it's hard for your body to turn these proteins into fat. In fact, it takes so much work for your body to digest them that you'll actually burn fat trying to digest massive amounts of protein.

How should you eat proteins? Again, fresher is better. This means that fresh chicken is better than the stuff you'll find in a can, bag or box. Fresh eggs are better than those to which you must add water. Yogurt is better than cheese that's been sitting in a package for months.

When should you eat protein? The best time is your last meal of the day. At night your body will break down the protein into amino acids, which will be transported throughout your body for much needed tissue repair. In the morning, you'll wake with a body that's ready for another day.

Depending on your activity level, protein can be good at lunch, too. Most sedentary people (especially office workers) will do well with a protein/vegetable lunch, which will keep weight off and help them think clearly through the afternoon. Physically active workers will want to add some carbs at lunch to sustain their energy throughout the afternoon.

The Skinny On Fats

If you've read this book up to this point you probably can guess that fats must have a purpose in our bodies, or else Mother Nature wouldn't have made them in the first place. So what do fats do for you? They play dozens of roles, from transporting certain vitamins in and out of cells, to allowing your nerves to transport electrical impulses, to giving you what you need to make hormones. Without fats, you couldn't live.

Unfortunately, it's hard to live with too much fat, too. It gets deposited throughout your body, including your arteries. It's associated with heart disease, cancer, diabetes, strokes and, needless to say, early death.

As in other food groups there are good fats and bad fats. Bad fats are found in greasy fast foods, diary products, red meat and many of the foods found in boxes and packages at the grocery store (the hydrogenated and partially hydrogenated oils mentioned earlier). Good fats are found in olive oil, fish oils, flax seeds, almonds and walnuts.

How should you eat fats? The best way to get your good fats is by using olive oil for cooking and salad dressing, eating almonds and walnuts for snacks, and taking Omega-3 fatty acid supplements. The reason you need to take these supplements is that it's almost impossible to get enough Omega-3 fatty acids from natural sources like cold-water salmon and sardines. You might ask, "Why would I buy fat supplements?" Because by taking in good fats and eliminating bad fats you will actually make fat work for instead of against you.

When should you eat fats? That really isn't as much of a question as when dealing with proteins and carbs. As long as you take your Omega-3 supplements, use good fats for cooking and salad dressing, and stay away from bad fats, you'll be handling fats well.

Cycle Savvy

By eating certain foods at certain times you'll automatically wring more energy from the food you eat. Your body has natural cycles. By honoring the cycles for taking in, breaking down and eliminating food you'll make it easy for your inner diet guru to create more energy. This is one of those "dieting secrets" that takes the mystery out of losing weight. So let's take a look at your body's natural cycles and how to use them to optimize your nutrition:

Morning: From 4am 'till noon is the time when you should be eliminating wastes.

Afternoon: Roughly noon to 8pm is a time for eating and digestion.

Night: 8pm to 4am is when you should be absorbing the nutrients from the food you've digested, using them to repair your body from the inside out, and storing energy for the next day.

When you wake up your body will have broken down the food you ate the day before. It will have the vitamins, minerals and other nutrients you've gained from eating the previous day, and it should be ready to eliminate the waste products generated.

Since your body should be eliminating food in the morning, it's best to eat something that's easily digested for breakfast. As we've seen, fresh fruit is the best choice. Loaded with good things your body needs to stay healthy, it's also the most easily digested food. Eating bananas, melons, peaches, nectarines or grapefruit for breakfast won't slow you down. These are also good sources of fiber, helping to keep your intestines clean and fresh.

It's best not to eat other foods with fruit. Wait at least a half hour before eating something else. If you can stick with fruit until lunch it is even better. Eating a mid-morning fruit snack helps keep your energy high. (Add nuts if you need more staying power.)

Another good way to respect your body's natural cycles when it comes to food is to eat your last meal early in the evening. Try to not eat anything after 8 o'clock. In today's world it's often difficult, but if you can finish dinner by 6 o'clock your body will be able to rest better at night.

So, to re-cap: A good basic eating plan is to eat fruit or oatmeal in the morning, protein and vegetables for lunch (adding carbs if you're physically active), and proteins and more vegetables for dinner. By giving your body the food it needs when it needs it you'll give yourself more energy and more nutrients for healing.

Handling Digestion Problems

If you want to use food to heal your body, you need a digestive system functioning at 100 percent. Using the energy eating etiquette guidelines above and eating the right foods at the right times—along with drinking plenty of water—will clear up many common digestion problems.

But sometimes you need more help. If you have problems digesting your food, such as acid reflux, gas, burping, burning, diarrhea or constipation, you can often heal your digestive system by using some simple techniques.

Combo Meals

One of the best ways to "de-stress" your digestive system is to stay away from combining foods that confuse your stomach. For example, meat requires your stomach to produce acidic digestive juices, while potatoes are digested with the chemical opposite, alkaline juices. Vegetables are "neutral," and can be digested by either secretion.

Because your body is intelligent, when you swallow a piece of steak your stomach automatically produces the right chemicals to break it down. But if you eat steak and potatoes, two opposite chemicals are produced, somewhat neutralizing each other. This leaves undigested food in your stomach far longer than necessary, consuming energy you could use for other purposes.

The best way to avoid this energy drain: Eat only one type of concentrated food (either proteins or carbohydrates) at a time. Some "bad" but common combinations are meat (protein) and potatoes (carb), fish (protein) and rice (carb), chicken (protein) and noodles (carb), eggs (protein) and toast (carb), cheese (protein) and bread (carb), and cereal (carb) and milk (protein).

The best food combinations: vegetables with either a protein or carbohydrate. For example, a salad topped with a chicken breast or spaghetti and a salad.

As you might guess, proper food combining is difficult for many people. For example, pizza is off limits (crust = carbs, cheese = protein), though most people would choose bamboo slivers under their fingernails rather than give it up. But if you suffer from indigestion, watching the food combinations going into your stomach is, if not the easiest, the least expensive remedy. It should be the place where you start to heal your digestive woes.

Try proper food combining and see if the benefits are worth it to you. A healthy habit: eat fruit for breakfast, which automatically means you'll be properly combining to start the day. Then steer clear of improper food combinations at lunch or dinner whenever possible.

Enzyme Enlightenment

If there is one supplement virtually all of my patients with digestive problems benefit from, it's digestive enzymes. Many top nutritionists believe enzymes should be the basic building block of almost everyone's nutritional supplementation program. The reason enzymes are so important is because they are needed for virtually every chemical reaction in your body. Vitamins, minerals and fiber will all be handicapped when trying to help your body unless there are enzymes available to help them work. Enzymes are especially important for breaking down food in the stomach, intestines and colon. Fresh foods usually contain the enzymes needed by your body to break them down. Cooking and processing, however, destroy these natural enzymes, leaving your body to digest them as best it can.

Powering Digestion With Probiotics

Other pieces of the digestive puzzle are the "friendly" bacteria in your gastrointestinal tract that complete digestion. Many people notice that after taking a round of antibiotics they become constipated or develop diarrhea. That's because the drugs have not only killed the bad germs infecting the body, but also the good bacteria lining the intestines and colon. If you suffer from constipation, diarrhea, or other intestinal complaints, you'll want to take "probiotics"--friendly bacteria that come in a capsule--along with your digestive enzymes.

Plugging Your Leaks

The lining of your intestines absorbs nutrients from food breakdown. It also acts as a barrier to keep harmful substances traveling through your intestines from leaking into your bloodstream. Over time the intestinal walls can develop small perforations. This is most common in people who take a lot of aspirin and other pain relievers, ingest harmful bacteria, or are exposed to a lot of pesticides.

When this happens bacteria, viruses and undigested food particles leak through the intestinal walls. Because they shouldn't have seeped through the intestine, your body's immune system springs into action. But things go crazy. The body begins turning on itself (an "autoimmune" reaction) and all kinds of health problems are set into motion. This condition is called "Leaky Gut". It's very common in those suffering from fibromyalgia, Chron's disease, irritable bowel syndrome, ulcerative colitis and celiac disease.

Supplements designed to help leaky gut strengthen the intestinal wall, keeping this immune barrier healthy so it can keep you disease-resistant.

Fiber Options

Your colon needs fiber. Think of fiber as indigestible scrub brushes that work their way through your intestines and colon, sweeping up clutter and gunk as they go. Unfortunately, because so many of us lack fresh food in our diets, our fiber intake is spectacularly low. After awhile our colons become slowed by sludge. In my experience, most digestive problems respond extremely well to fiber supplements. My favorite product is Isagenix greens (www. drbarnhill.isagenix.com) from Isagenix. I've seen a combination of this product, enzymes, probiotics and a leaky gut formula transform the lives of people who've suffered for years with digestive problems like diverticulitis.

Buffet Break

To summarize, oftentimes the easiest route away from digestive problems toward digestive health is to start taking enzymes and probiotics with your breakfast, lunch and dinner. In addition, drink the Fiber Greens product for breakfast. If you are still having problems, add a product designed to heal leaky gut, and practice proper food combining. This program works for the majority of people.

Detox For Life

Are you still having digestive woes even after using the above program? Or would you like to prevent digestive problems in the first place? Or how about this: Would you like to rid your body of toxins at a cellular level, returning not only your digestive organs but all of your organs to an optimal state of functioning?

To reap the above benefits you need to de-toxify. Why? Because we are being exposed to more and more toxins! Pollution, pesticides, second-hand smoke, bacteria, parasites, soda, preservatives, drugs—all these toxins can build up in your body, many of them being stored in fat tissue.

There are many ways to go about cleansing your digestive system while detoxifying your body. In my practice I look at the individual patient and what will work best for him or her.

Vitamins and Minerals for Health

No matter how good your diet, it makes sense to take vitamins and minerals. Vitamins and minerals are essential to life. They regulate your metabolism and help all of the biochemical processes involved in releasing energy from digested food. Unlike carbohydrates, proteins and fats, vitamins and minerals are micronutrients; because you need only small amounts compared to the other three.

Even though you don't need huge amounts of vitamins and minerals, chances are you aren't getting all your body needs from your diet alone. According to the U.S. Department of Agriculture, at least 40 percent of the people in the United States eat a diet that contains only 60 percent of the minimum daily requirement of ten selected nutrients. This means about half of us suffer from a deficiency of at least one important nutrient.

Think of taking vitamins and minerals as purchasing insurance for your body's health. You'll want to take a high-quality vitamin/mineral supplement each day. Some people make the mistake of taking single vitamins (such as taking a handful of different vitamins like C, E, and a B-Complex). But vitamins and minerals work synergistically, working together to produce optimum health. Taking single vitamins or minerals may not only be ineffective, but dangerous. You may want to take extra vitamins, but a balanced vitamin/mineral product should be taken in addition to any single supplement. National brands like One-A-Day or Centrum—or the vitamins and supplements you can buy at mass merchants like Wal-Mart, Costco, or your local drug store—are not in the same league as the top-of-the-line vitamins you can buy through health professionals. They contain lots of fillers and other undesirable ingredients.

Nerve Herbs

In the old west medicine men would travel around selling "tonics". These drinks were claimed to do everything from grow hair to cure blindness. While those claims were exaggerated, there are two herbs--Ginkgo Biloba and Ginseng--that are the closest thing to a tonic you'll find for increasing the overall vigor and youthfulness of your body and mind.

Ginseng

Ginseng gets its brain benefiting power because it's an "adaptogen," a substance increasing the body's resistance to stress and normalizing its functions. Numerous studies document ginseng's ability to improve concentration, memory and learning. Dosage: Quality counts when buying this herb. Most cheap products don't deliver benefits because of the special requirements needed to handle ginseng. Look for a product made with whole, unprocessed, six-year-old roots (ask your health food store or herb dealer for details) and follow package directions. Take the

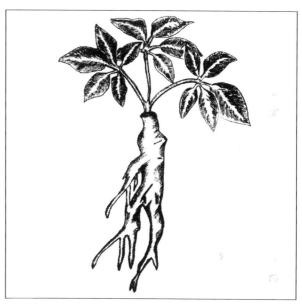

herb for a month. If you feel positive changes in your energy, keep taking it.

Ginkgo Biloba

Ginkgo improves blood flow to the brain and helps it use glucose. It's been dubbed an anti-aging substance because it seems to reverse some of the most common "getting older but not better" symptoms like decreased memory and impotence. Dosage: The herb is most commonly available in capsule form; follow package directions. Take this supplement for one month and note any improvements in your energy or thinking. If you feel positive effects, keep taking it. (Note: if you are on blood-thinning or blood pressure medications check with your pharmacist before taking Ginkgo, as it does affect your body's blood flow.)

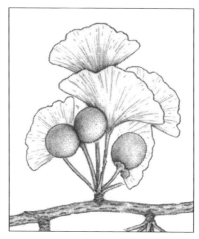

Super Nutrition

Blockbuster Supplements for Specific Health Issues

In the past decade nutritional supplements have been developed to the point where many of them work better and are less expensive than their prescription-drug counterparts. In addition, the products actually help the body heal, rather than just covering up symptoms.

These pharmaceutical-grade supplements may contain from a half-dozen to two dozen different herbal/vitamin/mineral ingredients, all aimed at helping specific health problems. Listed below are some of the most effective supplements developed so far. They can make a real impact on common health problems.

Adrenal Gland Support

You've probably heard the figures: nearly 80 percent of all health problems are stress related. Virtually everyone you meet today is "stressed out" to one degree or another. Your adrenal glands play a key role in regulating stress responses in your body. If they are overtaxed (and if you always feel "stressed out" they most likely are), your body will never be truly healthy, and the stage will be set for all kinds of health problems.

Supplements designed to improve adrenal gland function often contain: American Ginseng (helps the body cope with stress), Astragals (improves adrenal gland function), L-Tyrosine (helps reduce stress on the body; provides the building blocks for the hormones produced by the adrenal gland), L-Arginine (increases the activity of the thymus gland), 5-Hydroxy-Tryptophan (helps alleviate stress and nervousness), Vitamin B-2 (protects nerves and the adrenal gland), and/or Pantothenic Acid (an anti-stress nutrient).

Joint Support

If you suffer from arthritis or other joint pain, you need to take Glucosamine. How does this supplement work? It's a simple molecule that is rich in sulfur. The body uses it to build joint cartilage and other connective tissue. It also helps to reduce joint pain and swelling as well as increase joint motion.

There are other substances out there that have been touted as being good for arthritis. These include chondroitin sulfate, MSM, apple cider vinegar, and shark cartilage. There is no doubt that some people have benefited from taking these and other supplements. When compared to Glucosamine, however, they haven't proven to be as consistently beneficial. Once you get on a Glucosamine supplement, you need to give it six to twelve weeks to get into your joints and start working. You may notice relief sooner, but wait three months to see the full benefits.

Help For Sore Muscles

Combinations of the best soothing, calming herbs for muscle pain come in tablet or capsule form. They work well for conditions involving pain and/or muscular inflammation. They are especially good for menstrual cramps, traumas (like sprained ankles or whiplash injuries to the neck), and muscle pain from overuse (playing basketball for the first time in 5 years, gardening all weekend, etc.).

Their ingredients often include of Valerian Root (called "nature's tranquilizer"), White Willow Bark (alleviates pain and symptoms of inflammation), Skullcap (a sedative for muscle spasms that also reduces inflammation), Passion Flower (calms the nervous system), Bromelain (reduces inflammation) and/or Kava Kava (a natural muscle relaxer).

Natural Anti-Inflammatories

Inflammation accompanies other conditions in the body besides muscular injury or overuse, and it's often painful. Most people turn to drugs to make the pain go away, but with the drugs they always get side effects, too. Natural remedies are better, not only calming inflammation but giving your body substances with which to heal.

Probably the most powerful natural anti-inflammatory—one with lots of great health benefits—is Omega-3 oil. A combination of Glucosamine and Omega-3 oil is the simplest and most powerful supplementation program for arthritis sufferers *(see the "Arthritis Pain Relief Program" in this book for more details)*.

Herbal anti-inflammatories are powerful, too. They work best in combination with each other. For example, look for a product combining Ginger (a powerful anti-inflammatory), Turmeric (an antioxidant), Boswellia Serrata (a strong pain reliever), Bioflavonoids (these inhibit the inflammatory process) and/or Quercetin (a powerful antioxidant and anti-inflammatory).

Brain Food

The leading causes of decreased brain function are decreased blood flow to the brain due to circulation problems, lack of exercise, nutrient deficiencies and imbalances, hormone imbalances, toxic metals such as aluminum, mercury and lead, and diets high in sugar and other edible "pollutants". And like any other organ, our brains can get sick when we don't nourish ourselves properly.

Fortunately, natural supplements designed to increase brain function can make a dramatic impact on thinking and memory. These often contain: Phosphatidylserine (enhances memory), Carnitine (enhances memory and constructional thinking), Vinpocetine (increases blood, oxygen and nutrient supply to brain cells), Ginkgo Biloba (as mentioned earlier, increases blood supply to the brain) and/or Huperzine-A (improves memory, thinking and behavioral functions).

Growth Hormone Releasing Supplements

Do you want to be more youthful and vigorous? More "lean and mean," with more lean muscle mass? Do you want to sleep more deeply and wake up more refreshed? Then supplements that cause a natural release of growth hormone in the body are for you. Growth hormone plays an important role in bodily growth and repair processes, including lean muscle growth, fat burning, energy production, tissue repair, disease resistance, wound healing, memory, mental alertness, skin texture, sleep, bone density, normal cholesterol levels, sexual potency, and normal blood pressure.

After our teenage years, growth hormone levels decline at about 14% per decade. By age fifty, it's believed that growth hormone production may virtually stop. Growth hormone releasing supplements stimulate your brain to make and release this youth-giving substance. They may include pineal gland extract (helps support the pineal gland, which makes melatonin, a biological-clock regulator), anterior pituitary peptides (help increase growth hormone production), hypothalamus peptides (the hypothalamus directs the pituitary gland to produce growth hormone), L-Glutamine (a primary brain fuel), and/or L-Ornithine Alpha Ketoglutarate (an amino acid that helps release growth hormone).

Cholesterol Lowering Supplements

Natural supplements are fantastic alternatives to prescription drugs for lowering your cholesterol. They don't have the side effects of extremely powerful drugs like Lipitor, which are so dangerous that medical professionals urge people who take it to have their liver function checked every six months! Let me ask you, if you're on something that powerful in an attempt to fix your cholesterol problems, don't you think you should look for an alternative?

Some ingredients you may find in cholesterol-lowering natural supplements include: Beta Glucan (binds with fat and cholesterol to remove them from the body), Beta Sitosterol (protects blood vessels and reduces the chance for plaque build-up in your arteries), Policosanol (helps lower total and LDL cholesterol by inhibiting cholesterol syntheses), and Cordycepts (a hospital study of 273 patients showed cordycepts lowered total cholesterol by seventeen percent and triglycerides by nine percent while elevating beneficial cholesterol twenty seven percent).

Protein Drinks

The more food we eat in its natural state, the better. Having said that, there is a place for protein drinks. "Pre-digested" (meaning they are produced to be readily absorbed by your body) protein drinks with very little sugar (fructose, lactose, maltose, etc.) are the best. They are good meal replacements for those people watching their carbohydrates. And because they contain a complete profile of essential amino acids, the building blocks for muscle, they're great for body builders and others wanting to build lean muscle. This same quality makes them helpful if you are in a re-building process after a surgery or illness.

Another nice thing about protein drinks is that you can combine them with other ingredients. For example, in the morning, adding a couple of scoops of protein powder to your fresh fruit smoothie will help stabilize your blood sugar while giving the drink more "staying power," so you won't feel hungry before lunch.

Eating To Get Out Of Pain

If you want to tackle pain, begin at the table. By eating certain foods you can decrease pain-generating inflammation in your body. Also, you can balance your body's chemistry, which will quiet pain signals while giving you a chance to heal from the inside out.

The foods that prevent pain the best are fresh fruits, vegetables and certain fats. As Dr. James N. Dillard writes in his book, "The Chronic Pain Solution":

"If you don't feed your body well, it will not heal. Rebuild your bone and muscle tissue with the nutritional offerings of produce, or they will continue to degenerate and inflame. Feed your nervous system with fruits and vegetables, or it may be so weak and unstable that it sends out intensified messages of pain."

One reason veggies are so important when you're eating to get out of pain is that they create a basic pH environment in your body. You know that your stomach produces acid to digest food, but did you know that your bloodstream has a certain acidity level as well? If this internal environment gets too acidic it sets the stage for many health problems, including osteoporosis, arthritis and early aging of your internal organs.

The best way to create a more basic (and therefore healthier) internal environment is to eat veggies, veggies and more veggies. The most important vegetables to include in your diet are broccoli and spinach. Not only will they make your internal environment more basic, each is filled with B-complex vitamins, essential for a proper functioning nervous system. They also contain magnesium, which has a soothing affect on muscles. If you are suffering from pain of a long duration, being from arthritis or some other chronic condition, one of the healthiest habits you can develop is to eat two servings of broccoli or spinach each day.

The Acid/Osteoporosis Link

When your body senses that its internal environment has become too acidic, is will take calcium from your bones and dissolve it into your bloodstream in order to neutralize the acid. The stage is now set for osteoporosis. Many people think the high rate of osteoporosis in the United States is due to a lack of calcium consumption. The truth is that we have far more calcium in our diets than many other countries with much lower levels of osteoporosis. However, our diets tend to be much more acid-producing than many other countries. Sodas (which contain phosphoric acid), white flour, sugar, caffeine and meat are all extremely acid-producing. Our bones weaken over time as our bodies use them to neutralize an acidic bloodstream.

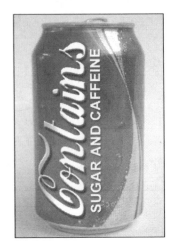

Besides eating vegetables and fruit, you must--especially if you suffer from tender, burning joint pain--watch what type of fats you're eating. Again, hydrogenated and partially hydrogenated oils will turn up the pain volume in your body, so use olive oil for cooking and salad dressings, which will help inhibit the formation of pain chemicals in and around your joints. As we've discussed, you'll also want to supplement with Omega-3 oil, a natural anti-inflammatory.

One last but crucial bit of advice when eating for pain relief: Stay away from processed foods. We've seen how these foods are unhealthy, but another reason to avoid them is that fast foods, white bread and sugary baked goods all generate pain-producing chemicals in your body. Even if you can't give up these items entirely, give them up until your pain goes away. In the end, eating right is one of the easiest and quickest ways to get out of pain.

Eating and Breathing for Energy

We've talked about how to eat and supplement your diet so that you're getting all the nutrition you need to live the healthiest life possible. But since chiropractic is all about getting your nervous system functioning correctly, I'd like to give you some other tools for working with this master system. Sometimes you'd like your nervous system to "speed up". In other words, you'd like to think more clearly. At other times you'd like it relax and unwind. By eating and breathing in certain ways you can accomplish these goals.

Diet and the Hyperactive Child

We've seen how eating affects our nervous systems. An extreme example are hyperactive children, often labeled "out of control" by their parents and teachers. These kids have nervous systems firing at warp speed. Their attention is scattered; they often leap from one activity to another.

Many children who've been labeled hyperactive are given powerful drugs to alter their nervous system function. A large percentage of these kids could be helped just as effectively by treating their subluxations and putting them on a diet restricted in sugar, dyes, preservatives and certain foods, and then supplementing their diets with vitamins, herbs and other nutrients to help their brains function the way nature intended.

The book, "Stop ADHD, ADD, ODD Hyperactivity/A Drugless Family Guide To Optimal Health" by Dr. Robert DeMaria (Drugless Healthcare Solutions, Elyria, OH (440) 323-3841) is a modern classic on this subject. Reading it should be the first step taken by any parent who suspects their children might be having hyperactivity issues.

First, let's look at how to eat and breathe to energize your nervous system and think more clearly: Your brain manufactures chemicals from what you eat. It produces two "alertness chemicals" and one that tends to calm you. So to think more clearly, you need to eat foods that create an abundance of alertness chemicals in your brain. You can do this by eating protein foods containing as little fat and/or carbohydrate as possible. For example, at lunch you might eat fish and vegetables. Of course, you can drink caffeinated beverages and supplement with Gingko and Ginseng to really boost your mental prowess.

Now let's talk about breathing. Without enough oxygen your energy will dry up, because your body uses oxygen to "burn" the chemicals obtained from food breakdown. Most of us breathe halfway into our chests, but to energize ourselves we need to pack air into our lungs. If you're like me (and most other people) you won't be able to breathe for energy all the time. It takes conscious attention, and we're usually concentrating on something else. The trick is to breathe for energy whenever you can. For example, in the shower, during your morning wake-up routine, during your commute to work, or when you go to the bathroom. Build it into your schedule so you're breathing for energy at least once a day, more often if possible.

Breath of Fire

This rapid, powerful, diaphragmatic breathing technique is an "energy tonic" you can use whenever you want to revitalize.

■ Sit up straight. Raise your arms over your head, thumbs pointing up (see photo at right).

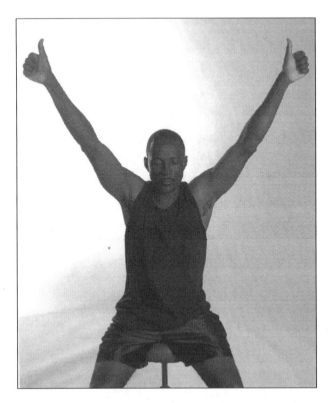

■ Begin by inhaling through your nostrils. Now, with fast, powerful exhalations and inhalations through your nose, breathe in and out as fast as is comfortable. As you do, you should feel your "belly" move in and out as your diaphragm relaxes and contracts. (This breath is also called "bellows breathing," because you are pushing your diaphragm down and up very quickly to inhale and exhale air from your lungs.) Two complete inhalations/ exhalations per second is a good rate. Don't pause between inhaling and exhaling. Continue for one to three minutes.

Eating and Breathing To Relax

Now let's say you want to calm down. Eating carbohydrates produces brain chemicals that slow brain function. That's why bread, crackers, muffins, pasta, potatoes, candy, cookies, pie, cake, ice cream, jams and jellies are called "comfort foods".

So, if your waste line allows it, to relax have a nice piece of pie or a plate of pasta. And you can supplement with Valerian Root capsules or extract throughout the day, or drink chamomile tea to keep your nerves quiet. How to relax through breathing? Your breath has two phases: The "in" breath is the energizing phase; the "out" breath is the relaxation phase. So calm down by emphasizing your breath's relaxation phase. Here's how:

Slow Belly Breathing

This breathing technique emphasizes the exhalation, or relaxation, phase of your breath, promoting relaxation.

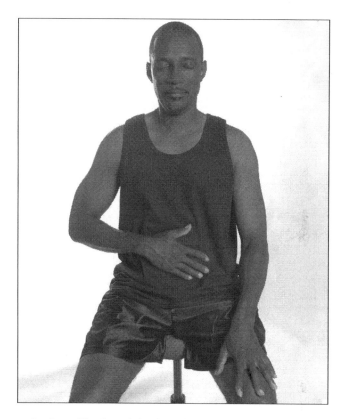

▪ Sit or stand in a comfortable position. Place your right hand on your belly, just under the navel. As you breathe in through your nose, imagine your belly is a big balloon you're filling with air. Breathing through your nose cleans and warms the air. Fill the balloon with your breath, feeling your hand getting pushed forward.

▪ Keep breathing in. Fill the middle of your chest…keep breathing, and feel the top of your chest expand. Now hold your breath for a count to four: "one thousand one, one thousand two, one thousand three, one thousand four"…then begin exhaling through your nose.

▪ As you breathe out, gently push on your belly with the right hand. Exhale the air at the bottom of your lungs first, then push the air out of the middle and top of your chest. As you do, count to eight. The idea is to breathe out for twice as long as you breathed in. If you can't do four seconds in/eight seconds out, try three in/six out, or two in/four out.

▪ Repeat slowly four times.

By following the basic rules of eating, avoiding nutrition villains, eating the right foods at the right times, getting your digestive system in order, breathing for health, and supplementing your diet with the right vitamins, herbs and nutritional supplements, you'll give yourself the raw materials needed for radiant health.

In the next chapter, we'll turn our attention to one of the most exciting aspects of the chiropractic lifestyle, the mind/body connection…

Medical professionals nationwide express confidence in chiropractic care

"Good medicine is about putting the patient first and chiropractors are an important part of the total healthcare team. Chiropractic works. I know this because my partner is a chiropractor, and I'm proud of that fact."

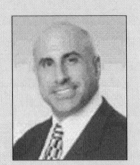

—Carlon Colker, M.D.
Your Health and Wellness Coach
Internal Medicine. Greenwich, CT

"Chiropractors are increasingly becoming important members of the traditional healthcare team, providing valuable contributions to a patient's health and well being. I can attest to this on a professional and a personal level. Following a car accident three years ago, I had the benefit of conservative chiropractic and orthopedic care and thus avoided surgery."

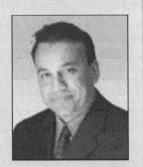

—Sana Khan, Ph.D., M.D.
Radiologist. Beverly Hills, CA

"I view chiropractic care as an essential component of our healthcare system. While conventional medicine does a good job of screening for the early detection of disease. I believe that the regular use of chiropractic actually prevents early stages of disease from evolving into crisis disease care management.

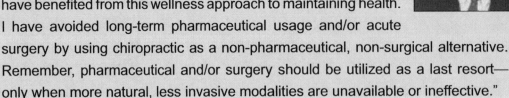

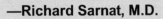

I have referred many patients to chiropractic care and they have benefited from this wellness approach to maintaining health. I have avoided long-term pharmaceutical usage and/or acute surgery by using chiropractic as a non-pharmaceutical, non-surgical alternative. Remember, pharmaceutical and/or surgery should be utilized as a last resort— only when more natural, less invasive modalities are unavailable or ineffective."

—Richard Sarnat, M.D.
President of AMI (Alternative Medicine Integration)
Highland Park, IL

7

BLOCK BUSTERS

[exercises & mental techniques for
strengthening your mind/body connection]

Heart Throbs

Trish kicked her right leg high in the air as the music pounded and the instructor yelled, "Do it again! Harder! Harder! Right leg down, left leg up! Right leg up, left arm out!"

Another 10 minutes of pulse pounding kicks, twists and lunges and the aerobics class was over. Sweat dripped from Trish's back as if from a faucet. She felt drained, and it felt good. Her ears still ringing from the amplified workout she thought about how tense her muscles were just an hour before and wondered, "Why can't my body always feel this good?"

Moving Violations

Hundreds of studies have demonstrated the value of regular exercise. "Use it or lose it" sums up why exercise is crucial if you want to live in a healthy, vibrant body.

If we use them, our bodies respond by working better. For example, if we take regular aerobics classes our hearts, lungs, arteries, capillaries and veins become really good at pumping blood. The benefits are astounding. Fresh blood delivers vital oxygen and nutrients to our cells while clearing out cellular waste products.

Weight training provides different but similarly sound benefits. Someone with more muscles burns calories faster, so they can eat more and maintain their shape. Muscle mass also has a great deal to do with physical stamina, our overall vigor and our ability to fight fatigue.

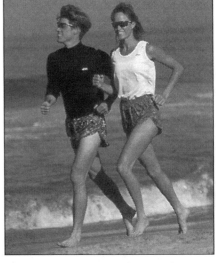

Not surprisingly, many of exercise's benefits result from its positive effects on our nervous systems. You may have heard of "endorphins". These are pain killing, mood elevating chemicals manufactured by the brain during exercise. They circulate in the blood, providing a natural "high".

Your brain works differently during exercise, too. For example, it starts thinking in a more relaxed manner 20 minutes into a 30-minute run, and keeps working this way after the exercise is over.

Exercise boosts our well being, too. Studies show running to be at least as effective as psychotherapy in alleviating moderate depression. In addition, our self-concept, short-term memory and intellectual function are all helped by training our bodies to work.

You Say You Want an Evolution

Most of us have experienced some of the benefits exercise provides our brains and bodies. But until recently few have considered how exercise can help the two work together.

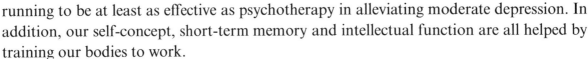

That's changing. During the Charles Atlas era and up until Arnold Schwarzenegger was winning his Mr. Olympia titles, health and fitness were associated with large, well-defined muscles. In the 70s that changed as the emphasis shifted to getting our hearts and lungs in shape through aerobic exercises like running. In the 80s and 90's cross-training developed, as a balance between big muscles and strong cardiovascular systems took center stage.

Perhaps because we live in a "stressed for success" society, today a fourth dimension is being added to the shape of shaping up, as the link between the mind, body and exercise becomes more clearly understood. As one women's magazine puts it: "Mindless repetitions are out. What's in: exercising your brain as well as your body."

What's emerging is a new field, neuromuscular exercise, referring to how our brains interact with our muscles and other organs to influence our well-being. The goal of neuromuscular exercise is to strengthen the connection between the brain and body, something chiropractors have been doing for over 100 years.

Most exercise will drain tension from our muscles. Neuromuscular exercise, however, is designed to change our alignment and relieve chronic tension patterns. After an aerobics class you can feel great, but within a short time you can again feel tension-filled. The goal of neuromuscular exercise is to change your body so those good feelings last.

It often feels like muscles have minds of their own. When our shoulders tense it seems like something inside the muscles is tightening up. But tension doesn't originate in muscles; it's rooted in our brains.

While it feels like individual muscles contract and relax on their own, every action of the more than 200 muscles in your body is controlled by the brain. In neuromuscular exercise you affect your muscles by changing the nerve connections between your brain and body.

Building Blocks

If you watch babies move you'll notice they are about as coordinated as a pile of Pick Up Sticks: the connections between their brains and muscles aren't developed. Our brains learn to control our muscles through trial and error. They weed out unnecessary movements, bit by bit moving more efficiently. As you mature you develop hundreds of habitual movement patterns.

Some of these patterns aren't healthy. For example, let's say you break your right ankle. As you limp around on crutches your brain automatically shifts your weight to the left leg, contracting certain muscles in your hips. A muscular pattern is established. Unless you retrain your body, the contraction may last long after the ankle heals. In fact, it can last until the day you die unless the mind/muscle connection is somehow "reprogrammed".

Surgeries can have similar effects, causing muscles to "cringe" in a protective reflex that lasts long after the surgical scars heal. Similarly, chronic emotional patterns can take root in our muscles as well: The overworked working mother who is chronically stressed can develop spasms in her neck and upper back as hard as golf balls.

As connections form between our body and brain our life histories become embedded in our muscles. Our bodies develop a tone--a state of relative relaxation or contraction--governed by emotions, traumas and mental states. These form an underlying pattern of muscular contractions influencing how we move.

Trish, our aerobics enthusiast mentioned at the beginning of this chapter, can wash away muscular tension with exercise. But her brain may tense her muscles again, resetting their tone based on her history. If she keeps doing aerobics her body will keep changing, as new movement patterns join the countless others in her brain. But she may never enjoy her level of post-workout relaxation unless she uses her mind to change her muscles.

Bring Back That Flowing Feeling

Up to now we've focused on how your brain sets muscle tone throughout your body. But muscle tone affects brain function, too. In general, **tense muscles make for tense minds. Soft, flexible muscles lead to flexible, open attitudes.**

Training to Stay Young

Power. Endurance. Strength. Flexibility. All of these physical attributes help to define our overall health as we age. However, as we grow older these qualities decline at different rates.

Flexibility is the first to decline, then endurance, strength, and, lastly, power. That's why a 50-year-old can lift about the same amount of weight one time as he did when he was 25, but may get winded walking a quarter of a mile.

Because the physical qualities that make up a healthy body change at different rates, it pays to put time and effort into them in the following sequence:

Concentrate on flexibility first. Stretching exercises should be done every day. Endurance comes next. At a minimum, you need to train your heart through cardiovascular exercises like speed walking, riding a bicycle, rowing, or doing treadmill work three times each week, elevating your heart rate to training level each time for a minimum of 25 minutes, with warm-up and cool-down time scheduled in the workouts.

If you want to maintain strength, there's no better way than working out with weights three times each week. These sessions need only take 30 to 40 minutes, and should include a workout routine for all the major muscle groups.

Power training isn't crucial for most of us as we age, but if it's important to you a personal trainer can design a power program that takes minimal workout time. By paying attention to the capacities of our bodies as we age, we can continue to be youthful throughout our whole lives.

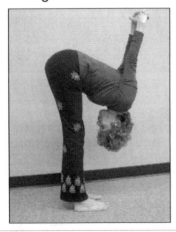 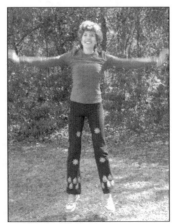 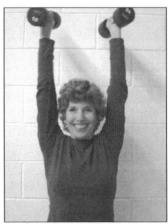

Block Buster Exercise

Certain movements and exercises reprogram the connections between your mind and muscles, releasing patterns that make you tight and tense. A great example are the movements/stretches associated with yoga and Tai Chi. These exercises get energy circulating through your body's "stuck spots"—those tight muscles and joints that just aren't moving like they used to. For this reason neuromuscular exercise is particularly good for the elderly, for those wanting better coordination, and for those who've sustained injuries that have never quite healed.

Below is a stretching/breathing routine, "The Dynamic Relaxer," based on martial arts exercises developed in China thousands of years ago. These movements are designed to move energy in your body. Like other neuromuscular routines such as yoga and Tai Chi, they are done slowly, with concentration. Here are some tips for getting the most from this and all neuromuscular exercise:

Move slowly

Moving slowly lets you notice tension in your body and gives you the chance to release it. Think about how, exactly, your body is moving as you practice each motion.

This practice of bringing your full attention to your body as you exercise is a key ingredient in all neuromuscular routines. For example, when you stretch a muscle you will reach a natural "end point" where the muscle stops stretching. This is your personal limit. Becoming aware of this limit and trying to expand beyond it each time you exercise is one of the main goals of a neuromuscular workout.

Thus, the end point of your stretch becomes your personal training ground, where you learn about your body's ability to go beyond its old boundaries. As you stretch, your mind fully focused on your breathing and your muscles, use deep exhalations to coax more give out of your body. Be gentle with yourself. Imagine the muscle letting go as you breathe out. When it does, smile, because you've just expanded not only your range of motion, but your mind as well.

Make your movements small

In traditional exercises we're often pushing ourselves to new limits (straining to run the extra mile or lift the barbell until muscle failure). With neuromuscular routines you will reach new limits by making small, slow movements that allow you to focus on what's happening inside of you.

Relax

Using a lot of effort makes it hard for your brain to notice what changes it needs to make in order to improve your mind/muscle connections. For example, if you've lifted a 30 pound dumbbell and a fly lands on it, the effort you're expending to lift the dumbbell eliminates your ability to feel the fly's weight. But if you hold a feather and a fly lands on it you can feel the fly--your brain is free to sense the change.

Rest briefly after each movement

Again, because your mind as well as your body is engaged in these exercises it's best to rest between movements or poses, notice any tension in your body, and release that tension before moving on to the next movement or pose.

Keep your knees relaxed

When standing and doing the exercises that follow, be sure to keep your knees relaxed at all times. Locking any joint in your body restricts the flow of energy through it. You want to stay loose in your ankles, knees, hips and shoulders as you move.

Tips for a "Dynamic" Dynamic Relaxer Workout:

Check your posture, breathing and mental focus before, during and after each movement:

* Your head should be lifted up toward the sky, as if a big hot air balloon was pulling it straight up. Your tailbone should be tucked beneath you, as if there were a rope at the end of it, pulling it down into the ground.

* You should be breathing slowly and deeply.

* Your mind should be focused on your breath and the movement of your body.

Eventually the correct posture, breathing and mental focus will become second-nature, and you'll be able to "flow" from movement to movement. But when you first start doing The Dynamic Relaxer you'll need to constantly bring your mind back to watching these elements of the exercise.

The Dynamic Relaxer
Approximate workout time: 10 minutes

The Dynamic Relaxer consists of eight simple movements. Each should be repeated 5-10 times. The whole workout should take 10-15 minutes. The best time to do this exercise is in the morning, before breakfast. However, the routine is an excellent warm-up for competitive sports, as it integrates your nervous system, helping promote peak performance. Get into a relaxed standing pose and begin the first movement:

Movement 1

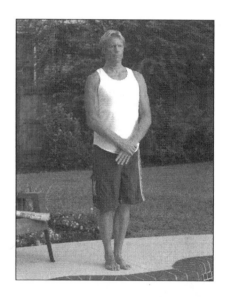

- Start with your feet together and grasp your left wrist with your right hand. As you inhale a deep, slow breath raise your arms, stretching both hands over your head as high as possible.

- Hold your breath for a count of two.

- Exhale slowly and let your arms down. (As in all the Dynamic Relaxer movements, inhale and exhale deeply and slowly through your nose.)

- Repeat this arm-raising motion twice to warm up and establish your balance.

- On your third rep, raise your heels off the ground as you extend your arms up, so that when your arms are completely over your head you are balancing on the balls of your feet.

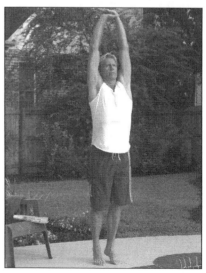

- Exhale slowly and let your arms down while you lower your heels. Repeat 5-10 times.

Note: If you have difficulty balancing on your toes as in the photo on the right, simply keep your feet flat on the ground during this movement.

Movement 2

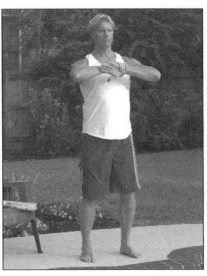

- After taking a breath or two and relaxing, spread your legs so your feet are shoulder-width apart. Grasp your left wrist with your right hand and hold them at chest level. Taking a breath, push your arms straight out in front of you as far as is comfortable.

- Exhaling, bring your arms back into your body to the starting position.

- Repeat 5-10 times.

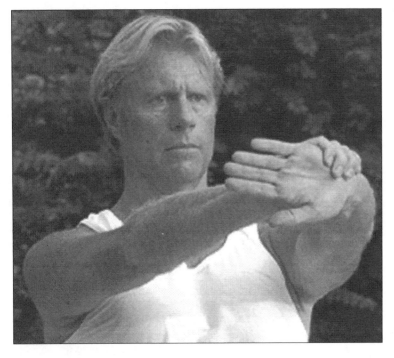

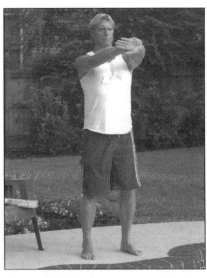

Movement 3

▪ Stand with your feet together, your arms at your sides, with your elbows slightly bent and your palms facing backward. As you inhale, arch your head and back so that you're looking straight up, and bring your outstretched arms up to shoulder level, rotating your hands until their palms face the sky. Your arms should extend straight out from your shoulders in a "crucifix" position. Move slowly to prevent yourself from falling backward.

▪ Exhale and return to the starting position.

▪ Repeat 5-10 times.

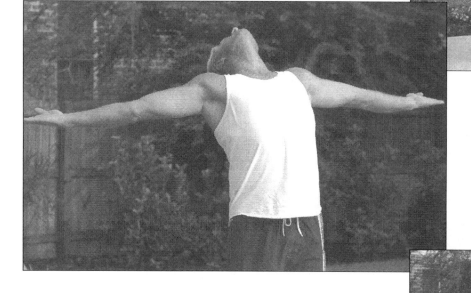

"The human body needs movement to balance right and left, to distribute and assimilate the energy, to circulate the blood and fluids, to prevent disease and aging, and to extend life"
--Hua Tou, Renowned Physician, 100 AD

Movement 4

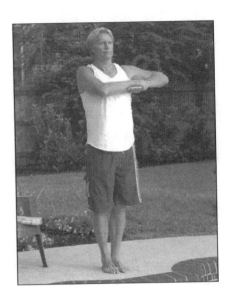

- Start with your feet together. Grasp your left wrist with your right hand at chest level, near your left armpit. As you inhale, raise your hands over your head, bending backward and to the right while you look to the left.

- Exhale slowly and return to the starting position.

- Repeat 5-10 times, then switch your stance and repeat on the right side.

Note: For beginners, start by standing with your feet shoulder–width apart, your left foot turned out slightly to the left.

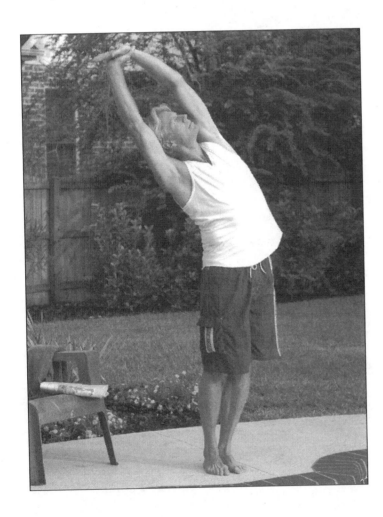

Movement 5

- Stand with your feet together. Intertwine the fingers of both hands so that the palms of your hands are facing up. Your hands should be at the level of your belly button.

- Inhale and raise your hands up to the level of your chin. Hold your breath for a count of two, then turn your palms down so that they face the ground.

- Exhaling, push your hands down toward the ground as you bend forward. Only bend as far forward as is comfortable. Keep your legs straight, knees slightly bent.

- Inhale as you bring your hands back up toward your chin; hold for a count of two then, bending over, exhale and push your hands back toward the ground.

- Repeat 5-10 times, developing a flowing motion of breathing in as you raise your hands and arms, holding for a count of two, then exhaling as you push your hands toward the ground.

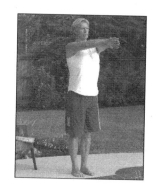

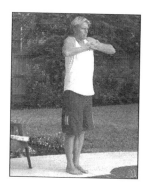

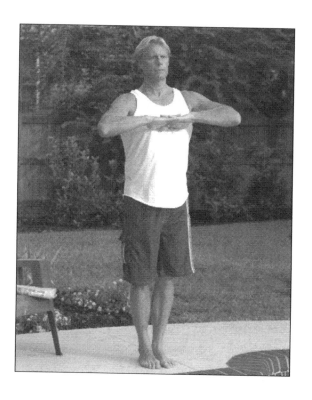

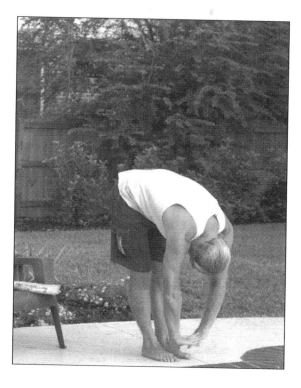

Movement 6

- Start with your feet shoulder-width apart. Make fists with both hands. Raise your left arm so that its elbow is bent and at a level even with the top of your head. Hold your right arm with its elbow slightly bent and your right hand just below waist level. Inhale a deep breath.

- As you exhale, slowly twist your body and neck to the right and look down toward your right buttocks.

- Inhale and come back to the starting position.

- Repeat 5-10 times going to the right, and then repeat going to the left.

Note: Feel a good stretch in your side as you do this movement. As you inhale, feel energy move up from the ground into your body, and from your outstretched arms into the sides of your torso. As you exhale, feel that energy expand throughout your body. .

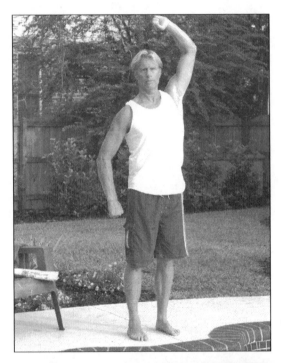

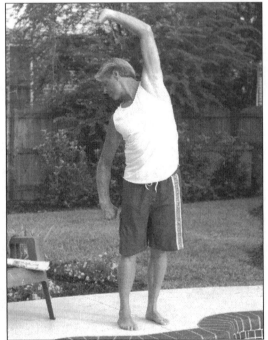

Movement 7

- Again, start with your feet shoulder-width apart. Hold your arms straight and slightly in back of you, with your palms facing backward. Taking a long, slow, deep breath, bring your arms in front of you in a smooth arc that brings the backs of your hands together.

- Exhale as you return to the starting position.

- Repeat 5-10 times.

Note: As you inhale, feel energy flow into your back, between your shoulder blades. As you exhale, feel the energy expand throughout your chest, back and shoulders.

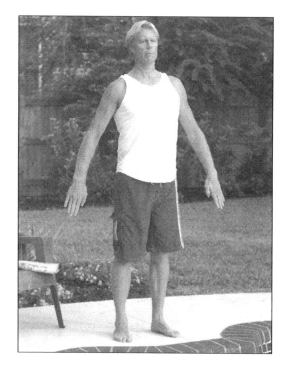

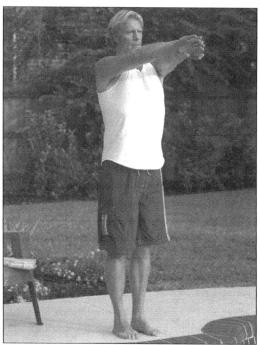

Movement 8

- Again, start with your feet shoulder-width apart. Raise your hands up to your chest with the palms of your hands facing the ground.

- Inhale and stretch your hands out to the left, keeping your palms down and your arms parallel to the ground. Stretch out as far as is comfortable while keeping your torso straight.

- Exhale as you return to the starting position.

- Repeat 5-10 times and then perform the same movements to the right.

- To finish The Dynamic Relaxer, stand still, with your feet shoulder-width apart, shoulders relaxed, looking straight ahead. Close your eyes. Take a deep, slow breath. Hold it for 10 seconds. Exhale slowly and notice how balanced your body feels.

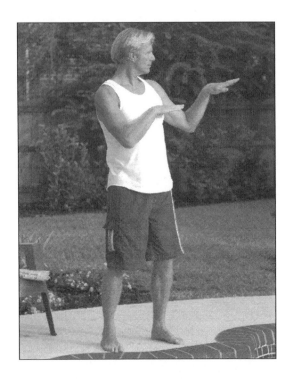

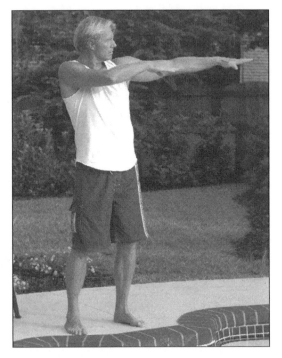

Mental Techniques For Relieving Mind/Body Tension

Thoughts can stream across your mind like clouds blown by a summer wind. They can also grip you with a heavy hand, demanding your attention. Behind the character of your thoughts lies their physical life inside your body. It's in your brain, over the vast fields of cells humming with electrical energy, that thoughts take a physical life in the form of tiny energy storms. Every thought is literally a flash of inspiration, a unique pattern of electrical energy in your brain.

But a thought's physical life doesn't stop there. The brain is connected to every cell in your body through nerves. When mental stress demolishes our peace of mind, physical stress results. As we've seen in past chapters, our thoughts have the power to round our shoulders and speed up our hearts. Because our minds and bodies are literally one and inseparable, we can use our minds to achieve calm bodies.

Mental Abuse

It's rarely the situations we encounter in life that cause our stress reactions. Most times it's our perception of the situations we find ourselves in that causes our brains to go into overload. A small annoyance can trigger an emotional reaction completely out of proportion to the situation.

Say you're running late to a movie. You throw on your clothes, stuff your keys in your pocket, and hit the road. Then you hit a traffic jam. Whammo! The pressure you were already feeling had sensitized your nervous system. All it took was seeing all those brake lights in front of you for your muscles to tighten, which may pull bones out of alignment.

I've had mothers tell me, "My children give me migraines. They start screaming and fighting and in a few minutes my head is pounding."

I point out that there are mothers who don't get headaches when their children misbehave. Something else is at work. If you get headaches when your children "get on your nerves," what may be happening is that your reaction to this stress causes muscles in your neck and on your head to tighten, aggravating longstanding subluxations, and your body starts to malfunction. It's pinched nerves and the resulting abnormal function of your body--not the screaming children--creating the headaches.

Wayne Dyer, the popular self-help author, likes to point out that if you squeeze an orange, what comes out is orange juice. If you squeeze a person by putting them in a stressful situation and they respond by becoming angry or nervous, that anger or nervousness is inside of them, not in the situation.

What causes your particular nervous system to tighten your muscles is very different from what leads mine down that same path. But both of us can decrease the chance of our bodies betraying us if we change how our minds work.

By using some simple mental techniques we can change the way we perceive stressful situations. Instead of coming up with new ways to deal with every stress in our lives, we can train our nervous systems to handle all stress in a better way.

In the pages ahead you'll learn how to calm your mind and affect the unconscious patterns ingrained in your nervous system. With practice you'll be able to calm your body.

You Be The Judge

The part of your mind most responsible for creating tight muscles is the one that is forever judging the world. This part of the mind takes the sights, sounds, smells, etc. it receives from the world, or thinks about past or future experiences, and then changes your body after evaluating your experience.

The situation where you're late for a movie and get caught in traffic is a good example. Your mind takes in all those brake lights. It feels you slow to a stop. It notes that you're going to be late. It then makes judgments about the situation that can cause your muscles to tighten.

It's difficult to stop your mind from these activities. That's what your mind does. The problem doesn't lie in thinking these thoughts. It's in being connected to them so closely.

Most people are so connected to their thoughts that it's impossible for them to separate themselves from them. It may surprise you that your thoughts are not you! It's possible to step back from your thoughts and let them pass by you as if you were watching a Thanksgiving Day parade and they were giant Mickey Mouse balloons.

If you constantly feel connected to tense thoughts your nervous system becomes like a rope being twisted tighter and tighter. If you consistently step back and observe your thoughts, you untie those knots.

"Our actions are all too frequently driven rather than undertaken in awareness, driven by those perfectly ordinary thoughts and impulses that run through the mind like a coursing river, if not a waterfall...Meditation means learning how to get out of this current, sit by its bank and listen to it, learn from it, and then use its energies to guide us rather than to tyrannize us."

...From "Wherever You Go There You Are" by Jon Kabat-Zinn

The Quiet Mind Technique

The Quiet Mind technique described below is a simplified version of meditation, the practice of which has been shown in hundreds of studies to reduce blood pressure, heart rate and muscle tension, as well as decrease anxiety and depression. It is the closest thing to a mental tonic you'll ever find.

In practicing this technique you'll sit peacefully in a quiet place for 10 to 20 minutes with your eyes closed, noticing how your breath moves in and out of your body, counting "one" to yourself every time you breathe out.

As we've seen, breathing is a powerful link between your mind and body. By focusing your attention on it you give your mind a break.

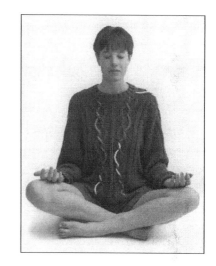

- Find a spot in your home or office where you can go at the same time each day to be alone for 10 to 20 minutes. The best time is the first thing in the morning, right after your wake-up routine and a few simple stretching exercises. Your energy will be fresh and your muscles limber. However, other times of day will do, such as at lunch or right before going to bed. In fact, if you have trouble sleeping a bedtime session is a good way to calm down.

- While not essential, it's best to practice the Quiet Mind at the same time each day because you'll be conditioning your nervous system to quiet down just by sitting in the same place at the same time. Sometimes your bedroom is best because you can close the door on the rest of the world. You should be able to sit comfortably. If you don't have a suitable chair or couch try sitting cross-legged on your bed with some pillows propped behind you. It may be too hectic at home. In this case you can walk or drive to a quiet spot like a park before or after work or during lunch to practice the technique.

- Once you've found a spot, sit comfortably, with your wrists resting on your knees, palms facing up. Close your eyes.

- Take a minute to scan your body for tension. Start with a deep breath in and then give a long sigh as you breathe out. As the breath goes out of your body feel your shoulders drop. Now focus your attention on your head, face and neck. Are there any tight muscles that could be released? If so, take a deep breath in and as you breathe out imagine that your breath is flowing out of the tight spot, and feel the muscles in and around the area relax.

117

- Continue scanning your body from the neck down. Focus on your shoulders, your arms, your chest, your upper back, lower back and belly. Then go down to your legs and feet. As you move through your body find the tense spots, breathe through them and let go of any tension. This body scan should only take a minute.

- Now focus on your breath. Notice how it flows into your body, hesitates a bit, and then flows back out. Your natural inclination may be to control your breath in some way. For example, you may try to breath deeper. Don't. Just watch the breath. Let it do whatever it wants.

- If you start to feel anxious try to let that feeling go. If your anxiety builds you can take a few deep breaths in and out, stretch your arms up in the air, relax, and then go back to watching the breath. If you start to feel really anxious get up, do some stretching exercises and try the Quiet Mind technique another time.

- Assuming you don't develop anxiety, as the breath flows out of your body silently count "one" to yourself. Repeat this process, watching your breath and counting "one" with each exhalation, for the next 10 to 20 minutes. If you don't have 10 to 20 minutes, do the Quiet Mind for 5 instead...any amount of time you spend practicing this technique is worthwhile.

- As you continue to breathe you may notice that your breathing gets slower and shallower. Don't be concerned. As your mind quiets your body quiets, too, and it requires less oxygen.

- It gets easier with practice. Within two to three weeks you should start to notice that you are feeling more peaceful.

The Wander Of It All

The Quiet Mind is a simple technique, but it may not be as easy to practice as it sounds. For one thing when most people first try it they are able to focus on their breath for only a breath or two. Other thoughts--the same ones constantly going through your mind when you're not concentrating on your breath--will crowd into your head.

You'll be sitting there watching your breath, counting "one" every time you breath out, and all of a sudden you'll realize that you're thinking about what you're going to have for lunch, or how your back feels tight, or how you need to call your mother...any one of a thousand thoughts will have crept into your mind, and you'll notice yourself following them, chasing after them as if you had a net and were chasing butterflies.

You'll realize that you promised yourself that for ten to twenty minutes you were just going to watch your breath go in and out of your body, counting "one" every time you let a breath out. You'll go back to watching and counting. Within two or three breaths you'll catch yourself thinking about filling up the car with gas or wondering if the bathroom needs to be cleaned...and so it will go for 10 to 20 minutes: you concentrating on the breath, losing that concentration to a thought passing in your mind, remembering that you should be counting breaths, and going back to counting your breaths until the next thought crosses your mind.

Other things may happen during your Quiet Mind sessions. For example, you may get sleepy. This is because your body has been trained to go to sleep when you close your eyes and relax. That's why it's best to sit up when you practice.

You may also find yourself thinking "worry thoughts". When you quiet your mind, all your worries get a chance to jump onto the stage of your attention. When this happens, and it will, you need to remind yourself that this is a time for letting go instead of holding on. It's one of the few times you can sit back and observe your worries from a distance, choosing to watch them rather than figuring out how to solve them.

You can also get anxious thinking about how bad you are at quieting your mind. "I'll never be good at this," an inner voice might chime. "All I can concentrate on is how good some french fries would taste right now!" It's natural for ideas to flow across your mind. This is the way your mind works. Don't fight it. Sometimes you'll be able to go for ten seconds before a thought takes you away. Other times it may be a full minute. The length of time between thoughts isn't important: Any Quiet Mind session is a good session!

8 Special Help

[techniques for maximizing your chiropractic care]

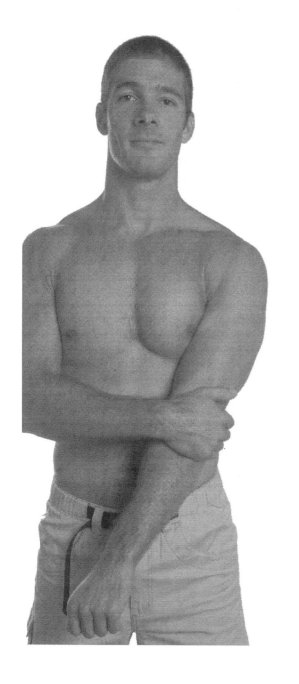

Help For Your Feet

Your feet are complicated, made up of 32 bones and held together with many muscles, ligaments and tendons. To work effectively your feet need proper nerve flow from your low back. So adjustments to the low back (and perhaps the hips, knees and feet themselves) are critical to getting your feet better. The techniques outlined below will also help. They are aimed at getting your feet moving the way they should and exercising/toning them so they can best do their job.

Using a Tennis Ball

- Stand with a tennis ball under your foot. Gently but firmly, roll the ball under your foot, searching for "tight spots".

- When you hit a tight or tender area, rub the tennis ball into that spot for 10 - 20 seconds, and then move on. Spend 3 minutes on each of your feet.

- Do this technique every day for two weeks, then as-needed when your feet hurt.

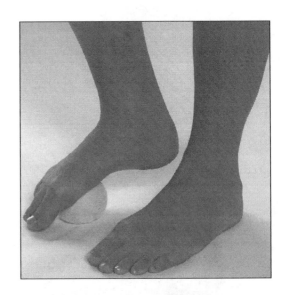

Using a Frozen Water Bottle

- Buy a plastic bottle of water and put it in the freezer until frozen. While sitting, place the frozen water bottle on a towel on the floor in front of you.

- Roll your foot over the bottle for 5 to 15 minutes. The ice will reduce inflammation in your feet, while the rubbing action will massage any tight spots.

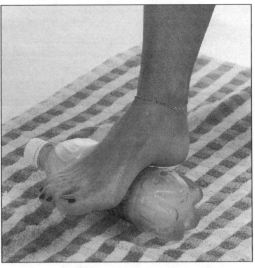

Stretching Your Arches With a Towel

- Sit in bed and stretch one of your legs out in front of you. Take a large bath towel and wrap it around the ball of your foot while holding the ends of the towel.

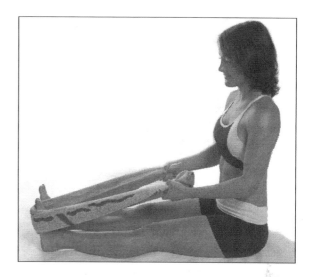

- Take a deep breath in, and as you exhale, pull the towel toward you so that you feel a good stretch along the arch of your foot. Pull just to the point of pain, and take two more breaths in and out, each time stretching a bit more as you blow the breath out.

- Repeat on the opposite foot.

- Do this every morning when you first wake up, before getting out of bed, until your foot pain subsides.

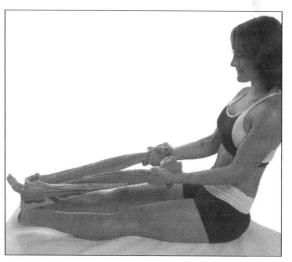

Note: Many people with arch pain are diagnosed with "plantar fascitis," or inflammation of the thick ligament that forms the arch of our feet. If you have arch pain that is worse in the morning (for example, if you step out of bed and get a sharp pain in the arch of your foot), then the exercises in this section will be particularly helpful to you. In addition, you may try wearing arch supports, such as the "Dyna Steps" made by Dr. Scholl's (available in most pharmacy departments). If these simple tools don't help your feet heal, custom-made orthotics made from molded impressions of your feet will usually do the trick. Also, many people find that wearing "clogs," like those made by Dansco Footwear, really help their feet feel better.

Scrunching Up A Towel

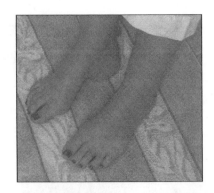

- Sit in a chair and place a towel on the floor in front of you.

- Place your feet on the towel. Using your toes, "scrunch up" the towel. This exercise strengthens the muscles making up the arch of your foot.

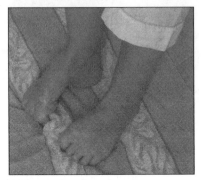

- Practice this for 2 minutes on each foot every day until your foot pain goes away.

Soaking/Pampering Your Feet

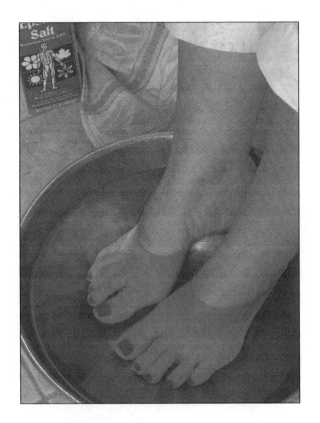

- Soaking your feet in a large bowel of water and Epsom salt is an age-old foot remedy that works well for achy feet (the high magnesium content in the Epsom salt is a natural muscle relaxer). In a large bowel place a half cup of Epsom salt and a half-gallon of warm water. Soak your feet for fifteen minutes.

- Afterwards, dry your feet and take a minute or two to rub a soothing oil into the arches, balls and heels. One recipe: add 12 drops of peppermint oil to four ounces of vegetable or safflower oil. Use one or two tablespoons of this mixture to massage into your feet after a foot soak.

Help For Your Knees

Knee problems are tough, because when your knees hurt they limit your activity, compounding health problems. By aligning the hips, pelvis and low back, chiropractic care allows the nerves flowing to the knees to work properly, allowing knees to heal. Adjustments to the feet and knees themselves may also be helpful. The following exercises also help the knees; they are designed to improve knee flexibility, strength and stability. These exercises should be done as a set once each day. **Caution**: *If you experience pain or swelling during or after these exercises, stop and talk to your chiropractor before proceeding further with your knee exercise program.*

Straight Leg Raises With A Towel

This--along with "Straight Leg Raises" (see next page)--are basic strengthening exercises for the quadriceps, the large muscles on the front of your thighs.

▪ Sit on the floor with your legs straight out in front of you.

▪ Inhale as you steady yourself and press the back of your left knee into the towel.

▪ As you exhale, raise your left leg six inches off the ground. Hold your leg in this position for a count of three. Now, slowly lower your leg down as you inhale. Relax for one exhalation then begin again, inhaling as you lift your leg off the floor.

▪ Repeat ten times, then switch the position of your legs and exercise the right quadriceps.

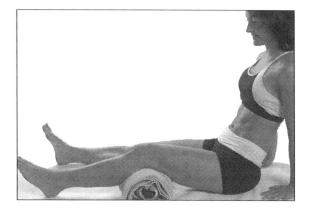 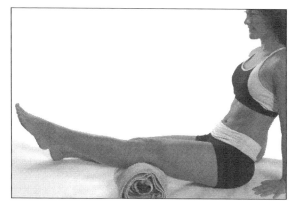

125

The Straight Leg Raise Two

- Sit on the floor with your legs straight out in front of you. Inhale as you flex your left foot toward your chest. Exhale and lift your left leg off the ground. Hold your leg in the air for five seconds, and then let the leg down. Inhale and begin again.

- Repeat 10 times, then switch the position of your legs and repeat the leg lifts with your right leg.

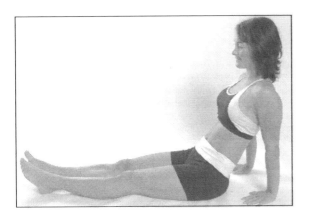 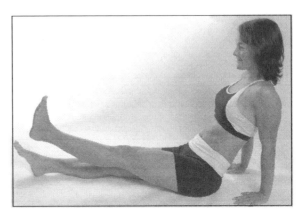

Leg Lunges

- Start by standing with your feet about a foot apart. Keeping your back straight, step out as far as you comfortably can with your left foot. Your left leg should be bent at a 90 degree angle. Don't let your left knee go past your left foot. The heel of your right foot may come off the floor. Hold for a count of two. Return to your starting position.

- Repeat five times, and then repeat the lunges with your right leg.

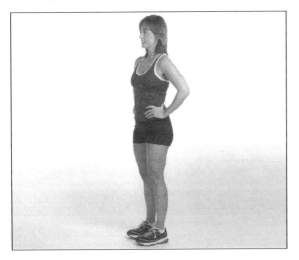 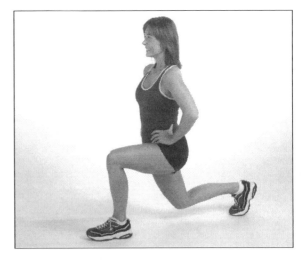

The Calf Stretch

Flexibility must balance strength in a healthy knee. Stretching the calves and quadriceps helps protect the knee joint from injury by helping to keep proper alignment and motion.

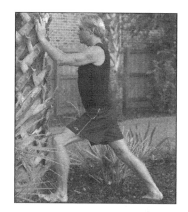

- Start this stretch by standing with both hands against a wall or other stationary object, elbows slightly bent. Your front leg should be two to three feet in front of your back leg, both feet pointing straight ahead.

- While keeping your back straight, bend your front knee slightly while keeping both of your heels on the floor. Keep your back leg straight. You should feel a mild stretch in the calf muscle of the straight leg.

- Come back to the starting position: repeat 10 times, then switch the position of your feet and stretch the other calf.

Toe Raises On A Stair

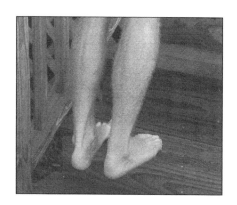

- Stand on a stair with your feet comfortably spread. Your heels should be slightly lower than the balls of your feet. Raise both heels, standing on the balls of your feet.

- Hold for 5 seconds, and then slowly lower your heels below the level of the stair.

- Repeat 10 times.

Note: If stairs aren't available, substitute a phone book. Place the phone book on the floor and proceed as outlined above. If you find this exercise difficult to do, don't use stairs or a phone book. Instead: stand about a foot away from a wall, using the wall for support. Again, raise both heels, hold for five seconds, and lower your heels.

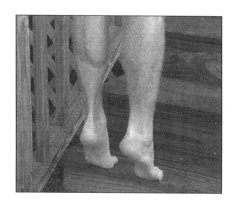

The Quadriceps Stretch

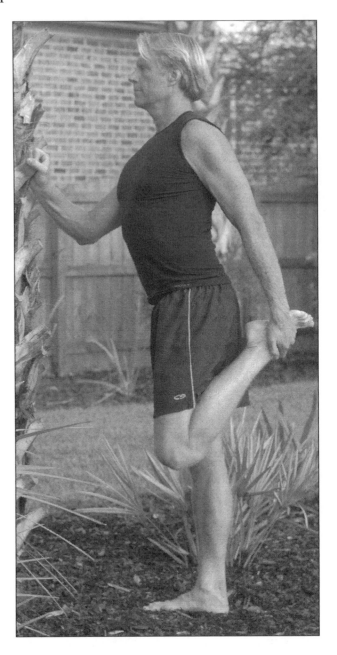

- Stand close enough to a wall so that you can support yourself with your right arm.

- Breathe in while bending your left knee, and take hold of your left ankle with your left hand. As you breath out, pull your left thigh straight back. Don't arch your back: maintain good upright posture. You'll feel a stretch in your thigh as you finish your exhalation.

- Breathe in as you go back to the starting position. Breathe out and repeat.

- Do ten repetitions, then switch the position of your feet and repeat for the right quad.

The Hamstring Stretch

Your hamstring muscles usually get tight when you sit in chairs all day. When they do, they can throw your low back out of alignment. To stretch these large muscles at the back of your legs:

- Sit on the floor with your left leg pointing straight out in front of you, its knee lying on or close to the floor.

- Bend your right leg and place the right foot against your left thigh, so that the right foot's toes are close to the left knee.

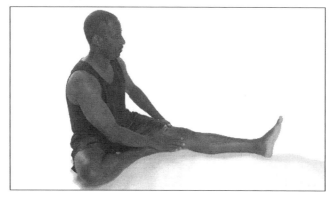

- Take a deep breath in and raise your torso up, as if a big hot air balloon was pulling your entire torso straight up toward the sky. As you exhale, bend your torso forward, toward the floor. Bend far enough forward to feel a good stretch in the back of your left thigh. Inhale as you come back to the starting position.

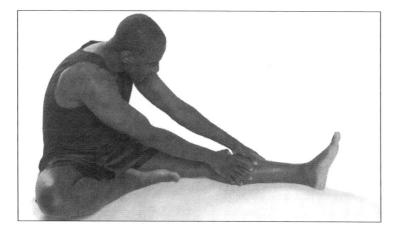

- Repeat two more times, each time coming a little closer to the floor when you exhale.

- Switch the position of your legs and repeat the stretch for the right hamstring.

    Note: Chapter Five's "The Bicycle" exercise is another great hamstring stretch.

Help For Your Hips

The following exercises are particularly good for pain coming from the hip sockets on the sides of your pelvis, where your leg bones join your hips. Remember, however, that many hip pains are actually caused by pinched nerves in the low back. Adjustments to the pelvis and low back often work best to relieve hip pain.

Squatting Hip Stretch

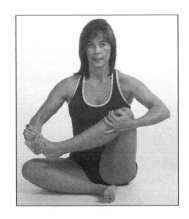

- Sit on the floor, cross-legged. Cradle your left leg in your arms (see photo). Imagine that your hip joint is the small end of a funnel-shaped cone, and that your knee is the large end of the cone. Using your arms, move your knee in a wide circle. You should feel a good rotation in your hip socket as you rotate the knee.

- Make five clockwise circles, stop, and then make five counterclockwise circles. Repeat with your right leg.

Basic Hip Stretch

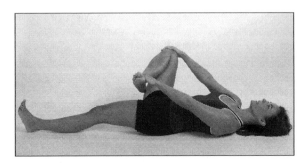

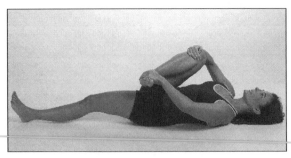

- Lye on your back; bend your right leg up toward your chest. Grasp your right knee with your right hand, your right ankle with your left hand.

- Take a deep breath in. As you breathe out, pull your right knee toward your left shoulder and your right ankle toward your left hip. If you start to feel pain, stop. Don't "pull through" the pain.

- Take five deep breathes in and out. Each time you breathe out pull your knee/ankle closer to your shoulder/hip.

- Drop your leg and repeat this stretch for the left hip.

Basic Hip Stretch Two

- Lye on the floor. Bend both knees so that your feet are resting on the floor. Bring your right leg up toward your chest and turn your leg in so that your right ankle is resting on your left knee.

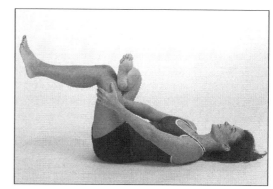

- Now bring your hands to either side of your left hamstring. Take a deep breath in; as you let your breath out, pull your left leg toward your body. You should feel a stretch in your right hip. Don't "pull through" the pain. If you feel pain, stop.

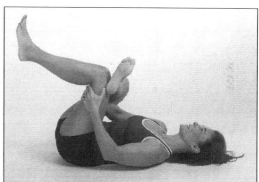

- Take five deep breathes in and out. Each time you breathe out pull your left leg into your body a bit more.

- Release your right leg and put both feet on the floor. Cross your left ankle over your right leg and repeat this exercise for the left hip.

Note: The Basic Hip Stretches outlined above are particularly helpful in situations where your pain seems to be coming from or centered in your buttock.

Hip Stretch On A Bed

This is a good stretch to do first thing in the morning, before you get out of bed.

- Lie on your back on a bed or couch. Inhale slowly and deeply. As you exhale, let your leg drop off the side of the bed and feel a good stretch in your hip joint.

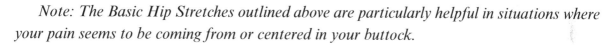

- Inhale/exhale three times, letting your leg drop off the bed or couch a bit more every time you breathe out.

- Change positions and repeat for the opposite leg.

Hip Stretch With A Belt

Note: this is a fantastic stretch for your hip joint. If you get "popping" or "clicking" in your hips, this is a must exercise. The key is to use a belt or rope to help you open up the hips. The belt lets you control the stretch so you get a little or a lot. This is an ideal stretch for athletes needing to add flexibility to their hips and back.

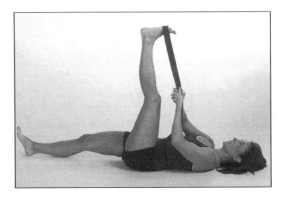

- Lie face-up on the floor, both legs straight and resting on the floor. Bend your left leg up and loop a belt around your left foot, holding the two ends of the belt with both hands. Take a deep breath in; as you blow the breath out let your foot flex and feel a good stretch in your calf muscles. With your foot flexed, take another breath in, and as you blow the breath out pull you leg toward your body, feeling the stretch in the back of your leg. Repeat two more times, each time bringing your leg closer to your body, stretching your leg out toward the ceiling as far as possible each time.

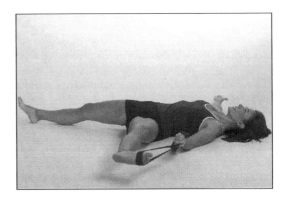

- Now, holding the belt with your left hand, extend your right arm out to the side at a 90 degree angle and let your left leg drop to the left, holding the belt as you straighten your leg and let it drop to the floor. (Note; you may have the let the belt slip a little to let your leg straighten all the way.) Once you are in position, each time you let a breath out let your leg and head drop further toward the floor. Repeat for three breaths.

- Come back to the starting position with your left leg extending up toward the ceiling and your head looking straight up. Take hold of the belt with your right hand and let your left arm drop to the side at a 90 degree angle.

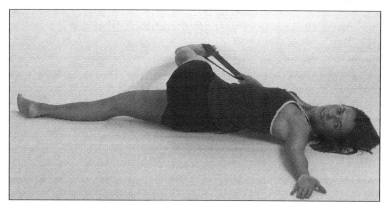

- Now bring your left leg over your body, letting it drop to the right, using the belt to help you bring your leg over.

- Once your leg is dropped to the right, twist your right hip beneath you and bring your left hip further up toward the ceiling; this should allow you to let your leg drop further toward the floor.

- Turn your head to the left. Once in position, each time you let a breath out, let your head drop further to the left while your leg drops further toward the floor. Repeat for three breaths. Come back to the starting position, switch legs and repeat to the opposite side.

Using Tennis Balls For Hip Pain

- Position a tennis ball on the outside of your left thigh by extending your left arm straight and placing the ball at the tip of your outstretched fingers (see photo at right).

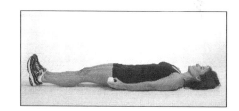

- Once the ball is in place, roll on your side so that the tennis ball "digs into" the muscles on the outside of your left thigh. This can be quite painful. Use your right hand to push down and regulate the ball's pressure on your leg. Hold for up to one minute, or until the ball becomes too uncomfortable.

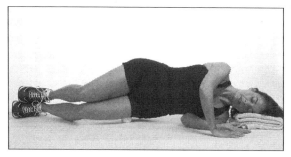

Help For Your Elbows And Wrists

Your elbows and wrists work hard, and because we use them so much they are prone to over-use injuries. To keep them happy, try not to keep making the same motions over and over with your arms or hands. If you have to do repetitive work, from time to time take a break and stretch your hands, wrists and elbows (see below). Switching hands whenever possible is also a good habit.

Basic Elbow/Wrist Stretch

This great stretch for the wrists and elbows should become a habit for anyone working at a computer each day. It stretches the muscles and ligaments on the palm-side of the forearms, and the tendons attaching into the outside of the elbow, typically inflamed from overuse (tennis elbow).

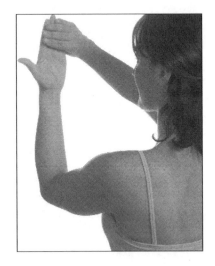

- To begin, hold your left hand up so that it's level with your face, palm facing you. Place the fingers of your right hand over the fingers of the left hand, palm facing out. Take a deep breath in as you raise your left hand toward the ceiling.

- Reach as far toward the ceiling as possible, and then—letting your breath out--curl your left arm out and down, using your right hand to bend your left hand down toward the floor. You should feel a good stretch in the wrist and elbow of the left arm.

- Do this stretch two more times, then repeat with the right arm. Do three repetitions of this exercise three times each day.

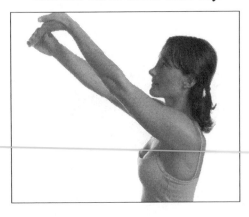

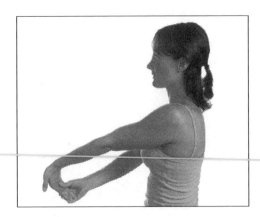

Why do we need to stretch the palm-side of our wrists?

Think about it: most of the time we use our wrists and hands to hold or grab objects, contracting the muscles on the palm-side of our hands and wrists. We rarely bend our hands backward. Over time, the muscles on the underside of our forearms become tight compared to those on the topside. This imbalance causes many hand, wrist and elbow problems.

Wrist Curls

- Start by holding a 2lb weight in the hand of the arm that hurts. With your palm facing up, lay your arm over your knee, with your wrist and the weight dangling over the knee's edge.

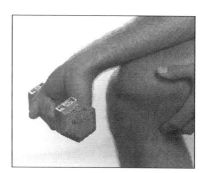

- Slowly curl your wrist toward your arm, and then slowly uncurl it. Repeat 8 times. Rest one minute. Do two more sets of eight repetitions.

- Do this exercise every other day.

- As you get stronger you may want to add more repetitions/ weight. If you feel 8 reps of 2lbs is too easy, work your way up to 15 repetitions. Once you can do 15 repetitions with ease, add another pound of weight, and go back to 8 repetitions, again working your way up to 15.

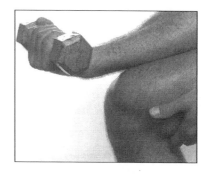

- Continue doing the exercise until your wrists and elbows don't hurt.

Note: If you are smaller-framed you may want to start by curling a 1lb weight. If you are muscular, you may want to start with a 3-5lb weight. The only way to know: if the weight you start with aggravates your wrists or elbows, go down in weight; if it doesn't feel as if it's working the muscles, go up.

Wrist Lifts

■ This exercise is done exactly as the wrist curls, but this time you hold the weight with your palm facing down, lift your wrist up, and then let the weight down again. As before, repeat eight times, rest a minute and repeat for two more sets.

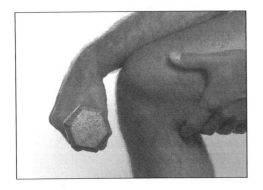 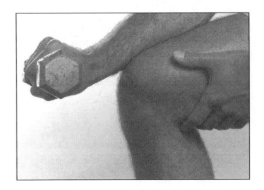

Self Massage For Your Elbows

Tight forearm muscles cause the tendons attaching into the elbow to become inflamed and painful. Massaging your forearm muscles releases tension from the area and lets your elbows heal.

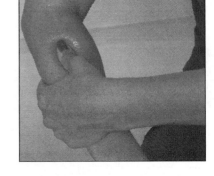

■ Begin by rubbing a small amount of vegetable or olive oil into your forearm.

■ Using the hand of the opposite arm, rub firmly into the muscles on top of the forearm, using your fingertips or thumb to look for tight spots. Work from the wrist up toward the elbow. You'll want to start by using long, slow strokes to relax the muscles. After a minute, use short, deep strokes to deeply massage areas of spasm/ tenderness. Work on these muscles for 3 to 5 minutes each day.

Warming your wrists/elbows before stretching, exercising or massaging them:

Microwave a hot pack until warm (usually one minute on High). Place the pack in a moist cloth. Wrap the pack/cloth around your wrist or elbow for 10 minutes, securing it with an Ace-type stretch bandage. Remove the pack/cloth. Your wrists or elbows will now be ready to stretch, exercise or massage, because the pack's heat will have loosened the muscles/joints and increased blood flow to the area.

Help for your shoulders

There is nothing better for stiff, sore shoulders than regular chiropractic adjustments. As with the rest of the body, shoulders stop working correctly when the nerves going to them (which come out of your spine at the base of your neck) become pinched. By restoring proper nerve flow to your shoulders, your shoulders can heal. Below are some stretches and exercises you can do at home to support your chiropractic adjustments.

Shoulder Stretch One

Do this exercise each time you take a shower:

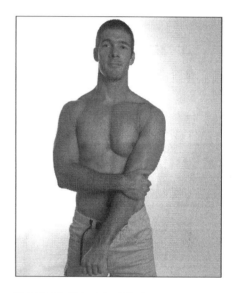

* While in the shower let warm water run on your left shoulder. Now, straighten your left arm and bring it across your chest, pointing it down at a 45 degree angle.

* Using your right hand, hold your left elbow and pull your left arm across your chest. Keep the left arm straight and low. You should feel a good stretch at the back of your shoulder.

* Breathe in and out three times. Each time you let a breath out pull your arm a bit further across your chest, all the while letting the warm water run on your shoulder. If one shoulder hurts more than the other, start with the sore shoulder, repeat on the opposite side, and come back to the sore shoulder once more, stretching it for three breaths.

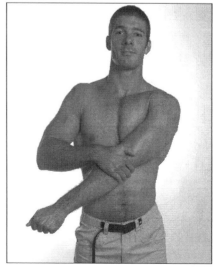

Shoulder Stretch Two

Now to stretch the front of your shoulder:

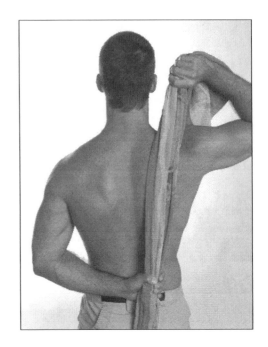

▪ Step out of the shower and put your left arm behind your back. Holding a bath towel with your right hand, let the towel drop behind your back. Grab the lower end of the towel with your left hand.

▪ Now, with your left arm relaxed, pull the towel toward the ceiling with your right arm, stretching the left shoulder. Pull to the point of pain, then back off a little and hold the stretch for three deep breaths in and out, pulling up on the towel with each exhalation, gradually increasing your stretch.

▪ Repeat with the right shoulder. Again, if one shoulder is more sore, begin with it, repeat on the opposite side, and then stretch the sore shoulder a second time before finishing.

▪ Do this exercise every time you take a shower.

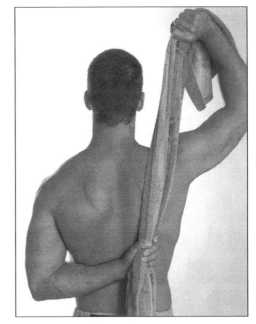

The Pendulum Swing

One big problem with shoulder injuries is that if your shoulder hurts to move, you consciously or unconsciously stop moving it. And when shoulders stop moving they start hurting even more. This exercise gradually increases your shoulder's mobility. I've found a good place to do this exercise is in your kitchen, at the dining table, but anywhere there is a chair will do.

- Stand by a chair that you've placed next to a table, holding a two-pound weight. Place your left knee on the chair to work the right shoulder, the right knee to work the left. Steady yourself by putting your free hand on the table.

- Let the arm holding the weight drop toward the floor while you keep your back straight (don't slouch forward). Take a deep breath, and as you exhale let your shoulder relax and drop down toward the floor.

- Repeat 3 times. With each breath you let out, let your arm drop further toward the floor.

- Now, breathing deeply and slowly, move your hand in small circles in a clockwise direction. Gradually increase the size of the circles in an ever-widening spiral. Do this for one minute, and then start over, this time rotating counter-clockwise. While this exercise is a good way to maintain shoulder flexibility, if only one shoulder is hurting you can save time by just working that shoulder.

- Do this exercise once a day.

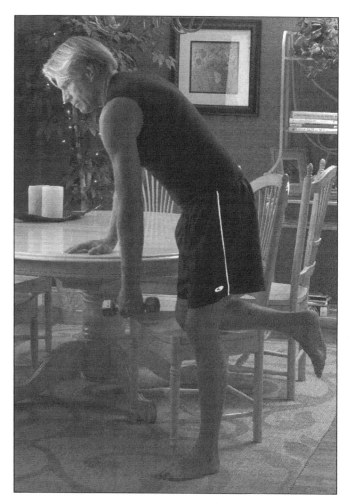

Wall Walking

This exercise is great to increase the range of motion in your shoulder. It's particularly important to do if your shoulder has become tight from being underused. A good place to do it is in the kitchen, using the timer on a microwave oven set for three minutes.

- Start by standing about a foot from and facing a wall. Keeping your shoulders level, place your hand on the wall in front of you at chest level and "walk" your fingers up the wall, as high as is comfortable. Mark this spot with a piece of tape. Slide your fingers back down the wall to your starting position. Continue walking your fingers up and down the wall for three minutes, each time trying to get a little higher on the wall.

- Now stand with your shoulder perpendicular to the wall. Again, walk your fingers up the wall as far as is comfortable and mark the spot with a piece of tape. Slide your fingers back down the wall to your starting position. Continue walking your fingers up and down the wall for three minutes.

- Each time you do these exercises try to "walk" a little higher, moving the tape up as you go. After a few weeks, stand closer to the wall to get more stretch. Continue with the exercises until you regain your full range of motion.

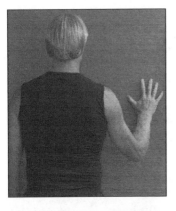
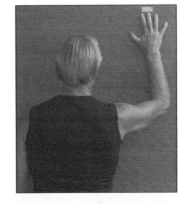
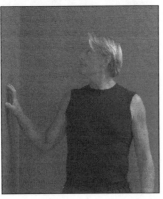
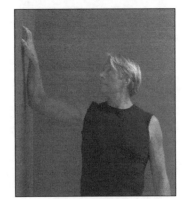

Rubber Tubing Exercises

Buy some rubber surgical tubing at an orthopedic supply house or sporting goods store. Take about 3 feet of tubing and tie a knot at one end. The knot allows you to "set" the tubing in a door.

- To start, put the knotted end of the tubing into a doorjamb at about the same height as your elbows and close the door (the knot will be inside the door; the tubing will be "squished" into the doorjamb; see photo at right).

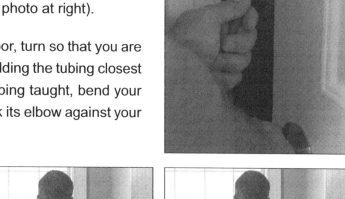

- Now, standing 2-3 feet from the door, turn so that you are perpendicular to it, with the arm holding the tubing closest to the door. Holding the rubber tubing taught, bend your arm at a 45 degree angle, and tuck its elbow against your torso.

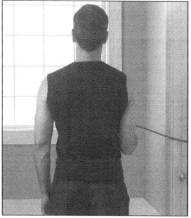
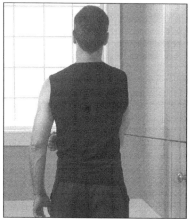

- Keeping your arm bent and your elbow against your torso, pull your forearm across your chest as far as you can. Go back to the starting position, and repeat for a total of 20 repetitions at a fairly quick pace, counting "one-thousand-one, one-thousand-two," etc.

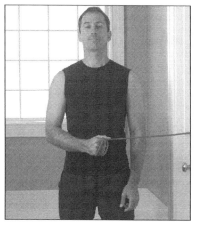
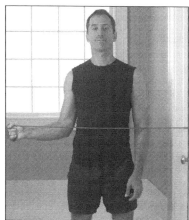

- Next, turn 180 degrees so that the arm without the tubing is closest to the door. This time pull the tubing out away from your body, again keeping your elbow pressed into your torso. Do 20 repetitions. Repeat these exercises twice each day.

Corner Push Ups

- Stand about two feet away from where two walls come together to form a corner. Place your hands against the two walls at about chest height.

- Keeping your back straight, relax your arms so that your weight presses you into the corner.

- Now push back out of the corner until you are standing straight again.

- Start with 5 repetitions and work your way up to 15 repetitions, once each day.

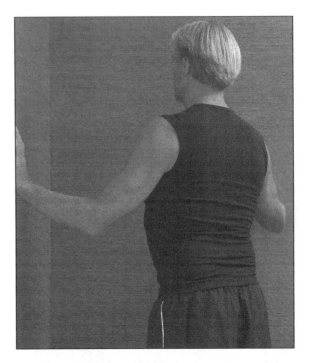

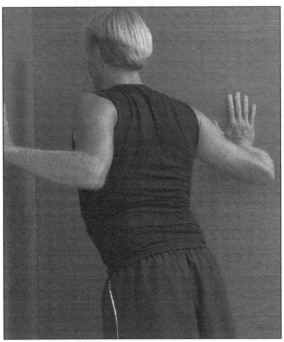

Using Tennis Balls for Shoulder Pain

Tennis balls work great to relieve the trigger points—small areas of muscle spasm—that often accompany shoulder problems. By relaxing these areas of muscle spasm, the surrounding large muscles can relax and resume their normal functioning.

- Begin by lying on the floor, knees bent, feet flat on the floor. On the side of the shoulder that hurts place a tennis ball at the back of the shoulder, to the outside of your shoulder blade (see illustration at right).

- Roll on your side so that the tennis ball presses into this area. Stabilize yourself by bending your knees and steadying yourself with your bottom arm. Place the hand of your top arm on the floor in front of you for stability. You can use your top arm to regulate how deeply the ball presses into the shoulder by pressing your arm into the floor (lifting your body up). Take deep, slow breaths and let your body sink into the ball. Let your head drop toward the floor as you let your body relax. This point can be quite painful, so be careful to ease your weight onto the ball, regulating the pressure with your top arm. The ball will produce an "achy" feeling. Continue to let your shoulder sink into the ball until the achy feeling starts to go away, which should be in 20 to 60 seconds, then roll off the ball. Don't stay on the ball for more than one minute.

- Now take the tennis ball and find a spot in the middle of your upper arm, about one-hand's width down from the shoulder (see illustration at the top of this page). Lye on your side and roll onto the tennis ball. Again, bend your knees to stabilize yourself and use your top hand to regulate the pressure with which the tennis ball presses into your arm. Feel the ache of the tennis ball pressing into this area, wait until the ache starts to go away (20 to 60 seconds) and then stop.

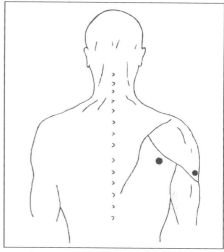

Areas on the back and sides of your shoulder where you'll work with tennis balls.

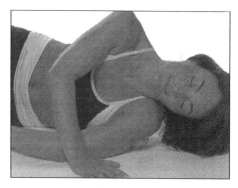

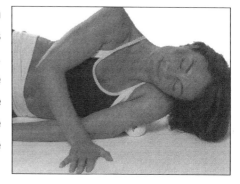

143

- Now move to the front of your shoulder. You'll be working on an acupressure point associated with tight pectoral muscles (the large muscles on the front of your chest). While you can use a tennis ball to work on this spot, it's easier to use your fingers.

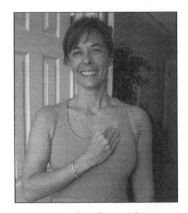

- Find the spot by bringing your fingers to where the end of your collarbone joins your shoulder. Come straight down your chest about the width of your hand. Press into this area with your fingers until you find the most tender spot (see photo at right). Press into this area firmly. You should feel an "achy" kind of pain. Press firmly for 20-60 seconds, until the achy sensation starts to go away.

Area on the front of your chest you'll want to work for shoulder problems.

- If you have the time, work on the three spots outlined above 3-4 times each day until your shoulder pain improves. If time doesn't permit this, work on the spots once each day along with your other shoulder work.

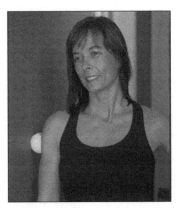

- If you find it difficult to do this work on the floor, try using a wall. Place the tennis ball on the wall and lean your body against it, feeling the ache for 20-60 seconds until it begins to fade. This works for both the point outside the shoulder blade and the point in the center of the upper arm.

Note: As a general guideline, when working on trigger points using tennis balls you want to feel an "achy" pain, but you don't want to produce sensations that are really painful. Since pain is a very personal experience, it's difficult to tell you the exact amount of pressure to use. My best advice is to go slow, using less pressure at first and building up as time goes on. Also, when doing this technique you will probably not experience a total cessation of pain. You only want to stay on the ball until the achy feeling starts to go away (say, when it goes from a ten down to a seven or eight).

Threading the Needle

This is a great stretch to do after you've finished your other shoulder work. It seems to integrate your shoulder's new flexibility into your body.

- Begin in the "table position" on your hands and knees, your back flat and parallel with the floor.

- Bring your right arm off the floor and straighten your right hand so that your fingers are together and your fingers, wrist and forearm are all straight and in alignment with each other.

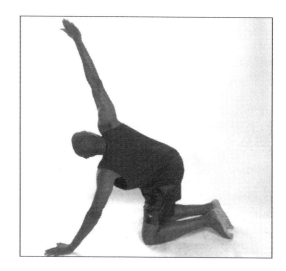

- Take a deep breath in as you raise your right arm out and up, twisting your body to the right and looking up and over your right shoulder, toward the ceiling. Feel the stretch from your armpit to the tips of your fingers as you look up toward the ceiling and stretch. Hold the position while you take a breath in, breathe out, and take another breath in.

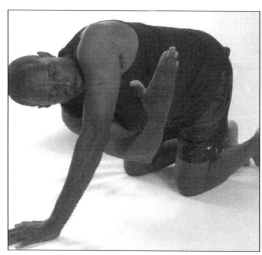

- Now, as you breathe out, bring your arm down and across your chest, stretching your arm as far to the left as is comfortable while twisting your body and looking left. Hold the stretch for five seconds.

- Repeat four times, then stretch the left shoulder.

Help For Your Headaches

Chiropractic adjustments are the treatment of choice for headache sufferers. Literally hundreds of thousands of people over the years have finally had their headaches go away after seeing a chiropractor. The following advice can be helpful in those extremely difficult cases where additional factors keep causing your body to go out of adjustment.

Dietary Factors

Sometimes the foods you eat can be involved in your headaches. Most experts agree that you should avoid milk and diary products. These are some of the most headache-producing foods around. Other foods known to cause headaches in some people are wheat products, oranges, eggs, corn, plums, raspberries, fatty or fried foods and onions. In addition, alcohol, chocolate and sugary sweets bring on head pounding in many, as do sodas, coffee and other drinks containing caffeine.

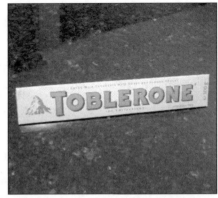

To find out if foods are contributing to your headaches you'll need to use a rotation diet, in which you stop eating certain foods for several weeks, note the frequency and severity of your headaches, and then re-introduce the foods back into your diet. For more information on designing a plan for yourself see, "Overcoming Allergies: Home Remedies—Elimination and Rotation Diets—Complimentary Therapies" by Christina Scott-Moncrieff.

No matter what your diet, drinking 8-10 glasses of distilled water each day helps most people reduce their headache problems.

Relaxation and Exercise

Since stress can be a major factor in your susceptibility to headaches, you need to "stress proof" your body. This best way to do this is to get regular exercise and practice a meditation technique. At a minimum, take a 25-minute walk three times each week. Practice a meditation technique for 10-20 minutes each day, as your schedule permits.

Trigger Point Work

The "Trigger Fingers" and "Trigger Fingers With A Partner" exercises in this book are excellent tools to soften the spasmodic muscles in the neck that often trigger headache pain. If done on a consistent basis these techniques give great results.

Use Ice Water

Because blood vessels and muscles respond to temperature changes, you can often use extreme temperatures to get headaches to loosen their grip on you.

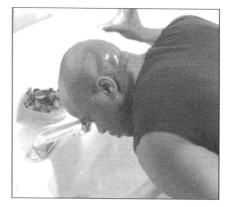

Fill a container with a quart of ice water. Stand with your head bowed over a sink. Place the container at the base of your skull, and let the cold water run onto your head so that it flows under your hair and drips off of your forehead into the sink. Pour the water out slowly and steadily, so that it takes about a minute to empty the quart container. Follow this by filling the container with ice water again, this time pouring the water over the soles of your feet for one minute.

Similarly, applying an ice pack to your forehead for five to ten minutes can often provide headache relief.

Use Pressure

Pressure applied to your head can change how the blood vessels and muscles on your head are functioning, perhaps short-circuiting headache pain.

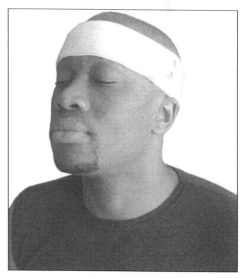

The easiest way to "pressure" your headaches into leaving is to take the heels of your hands and press them into the sides of your temples as hard as you can, pressing for as long as you can. When you get tired, slowly release the pressure. Hopefully your headache will have faded.

Similarly, you can take an Ace-type elastic bandage and wrap it tightly around your head. Again, some people swear by this simple technique.

Put On Peppermint

An easy and fragrant solution to tension headaches: Buy peppermint essential oil from a health food store. When you notice a headache coming on, rub the oil into your temples and forehead. One study found this trick as helpful as taking acetaminophen, a common over-the-counter pain reliever.

Boost Your Magnesium

Low levels of magnesium are associated with tension and migraine headaches, probably because a magnesium deficiency will trigger muscle spasms. So try taking magnesium supplements and see if your headaches are less frequent or severe.

Help For Your Jaws

The TMJ's (temporal mandibular joints) are the most-used joints in the body. Surprisingly to most, these joints are at the root of many health problems. TMJ dysfunction is most associated with headaches, neck pain and, of course, jaw pain. But when this joint isn't working correctly it can cause problems ranging from ear infections to balance problems. Chiropractic adjustments to the neck will often get the TMJ's working again. There are also adjustments for the jaw itself that re-align it and restore its proper motion. The techniques listed here will help your jaw joints heal so they can continue to work hard for you.

Hot Pack Therapy

Note: Do this before the other techniques outlined below. The heat will help loosen your facial muscles, improving your results when you stretch or massage your jaw.

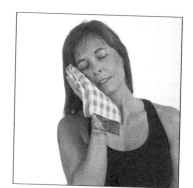

- Take a hot pack and wrap it in a moist dishtowel. Heat the pack/towel in a microwave oven for forty-five seconds to one minute. The pack/towel should be nice and warm, but comfortable to hold in your hands.

- Place the pack/towel against your jaw and hold it there for 10-15 minutes.

- Repeat on the other side of your jaw.

Pterygoid Massage

This massage can be quite painful. Go easy on yourself, gradually increasing the pressure as you press in on this tough muscle.

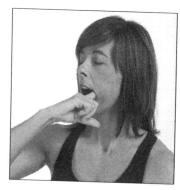

- Open your mouth and, using the tip of your index finger, reach into your mouth and find the spot where your upper and lower jaws meet (the space between your upper and lower teeth, at the back of your mouth). This is your pterygoid muscle, and if you have TMJ problems, it will be tight and painful to the touch.

■ Using the tip of your finger, gradually apply pressure to the pterygoid, pushing straight back. Stop pushing when you feel pain.

■ Now take deep, slow breaths, and every time you let a breath out, push back a little more and move your finger up and down, massaging the pterygoid. Massage for one minute, and then repeat on the other side. If your TMJ is bothering you do this massage three times each day.

Pressure Points For Jaw Pain

■ Start by placing your thumbs where your cheekbones join your nose (see illustration).

■ Press into the muscles right beneath the cheekbones while you open your bottom jaw completely. You'll want to press the thumbs up into the undersides of your jaws. You may experience pain. That's O.K. Continue pressing into the muscles while pushing your lower jaw toward the floor. The pain should start to lessen in 10 to 30 seconds. Once the pain starts to go away (say it goes from a "10" to a "7"), move your thumbs one thumb's-width out toward your ears. Repeat the process of pressing in with your thumbs while you push your lower jaw toward the floor. Again, once the pain starts to go away, move your thumbs out and repeat again.

■ Once you get out toward the TMJ's you may feel more pain. Just keep going until you've worked the entire underside of your cheekbones. Do this routine three times each day when your TMJ is bothering you.

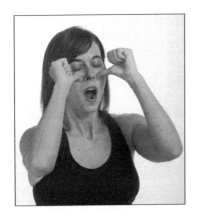 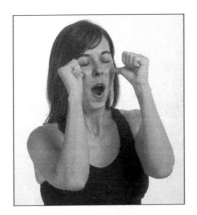 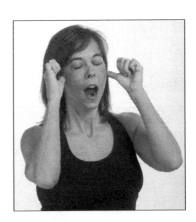

Help For Your Sinuses

Sinus problems are common. Chiropractic adjustments are especially good for clearing up even the toughest sinus conditions. Here are some helpful techniques you can do at home to supplement your chiropractic care:

The Magic Of The Neti Pot

One of the very best things you can do for your sinuses is to wash them regularly with salt water. A Neti Pot—a small vessel that looks like a miniature genie pot—can do wonders:

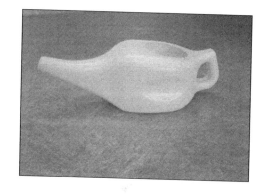

- Fill the pot with warm salt water (one teaspoon of salt to a quart of water). Position your head to allow water to flow through your nose: Lean over a sink and, holding the Neti pot in your right hand, insert the spout into your right nostril. It should form a seal so water won't leak out. Now, bend your head to the left, so that your right nostril is directly above your left nostril. Your forehead should remain higher than your chin. Raise the handle of the Neti pot so the salt water enters into the right nostril. In a few seconds it will begin to drain out the left nostril and into the sink. As you are cleaning your nostrils breathe through your mouth. This will help to keep the salt water from running down into your throat

- When the Neti pot is empty, exhale through both nostrils to clear them of excess mucus, and then gently blow your nose into a tissue. Fill the Neti pot and repeat the process on the left side. To order a Neti pot like the one pictured here, which comes with prepared salt solution packets and instructions, go to www.sinucleanse.com.

- For chronic problems you should flush your sinuses twice a day until your condition clears, then several times a week to keep them free flowing.

Breathing Easier With Acupressure

Several acupressure points on the face can be stimulated to help open your sinuses and keep them open. Here's what to do:

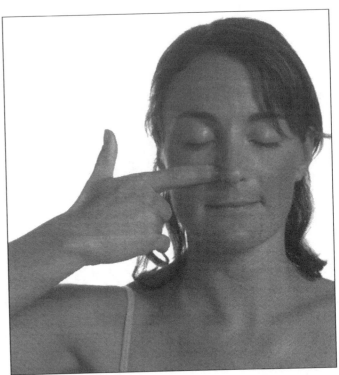

- Take the index finger of your right hand and place the tip of the finger at the base of your nose. You should feel a small indentation in the bone at that point, almost as if it were made to fit the tip of your finger. Firmly apply pressure to this indentation while rotating your finger counter clockwise for 30 seconds (traditional Chinese acupressure suggest rubbing 81 times—which takes about 30 seconds).

- Now for the left sinuses: Use the tip of your left index finger and rotate for 30 seconds in a *clockwise* direction.

- You should feel an immediate opening of clogged sinuses. The more you do the technique, the longer lasting the results. A good place to do this acupressure technique is in the shower, where the warm, moist air will help to open the sinuses as well.

Help For Your Arthritis

40 million Americans—one in seven people—suffer with some form of arthritis.

Most take drugs such as aspirin, ibuprofen, Aleve, Motrin, Tylenol or Celebrex to help them with their pain. These drugs are called NSAID's (non-steroidal anti-inflammatory drugs). They all have side effects. Most either cause gastrointestinal bleeding or put a strain on the kidneys and liver. Some of these chemicals interfere with normal cartilage formation, so that as they are relieving pain they are causing your joints to wear our quicker. For example, clinical research shows that Naproxsyn (Aleve) and Celebrex cause hip joint deterioration and speed up the need for hip replacement surgery!

More serious side effects include stomach ulcers, hypertension, congestive heart failure, and kidney failure. (Did you know that over 500 people die each year in the U.S. due to Tylenol overdoses alone?)

There is a better way to handle your arthritis.

Life is motion. So the first step in healing arthritis is getting your joints moving. Conservative chiropractic care is the best way to increase joint mobility and align the body so abnormal stresses don't contribute to further joint degeneration. But how to handle the pain? Over the last decade research has proven that a regimen of nutritional supplements does as good as NSAID's at relieving common arthritis pain. Not only that, in many cases these supplements can stop and even reverse the progression of arthritis.

Following is the latest information on nutritional supplements for healing arthritis. It's followed by a 9-step program. The result of years of research and testing, this program is the best way to heal your arthritis.

Glucosamine Sulfate

Glucosamine sulfate was first used to treat creaky bones in horses and dogs. Now millions of Americans take this supplement to give themselves healthier joints. Glucosamine inhibits the breakdown of joint cartilage. It also hydrates cartilage while stimulating its growth. The bottom line: Taking glucosamine helps keep your joints moist, springy, smooth and slippery. The best formulations combine glucosamine with other joint-healing ingredients.

Omega −3 Fatty Acids

Omega-3 oil is a fatty acid that reduces joint inflammation. This nutrient is found naturally in flaxseeds, walnuts and oily fish like salmon and mackerel. The easiest way to get your daily dose, however, is by taking Omega-3 oil as a supplement in capsule form.

Enzyme Supplements

When joints swell, it's largely because the fluids in and around them become infiltrated with protein-rich fluids. These slow the lymphatic drainage system, causing congestion. Plant enzymes in supplement form break down these proteins, facilitating lymphatic drainage, relieving swollen, stiff joints. Enzyme supplements containing Bromelain (from pineapple) and papain (from papaya) are best at reducing swelling.

Pain Relief Ointments

Pain-relieving topical ointments absorb through the skin to help relieve inflammation. In my experience the product Biofreeze works best for most people. It works great, feels cool when applied, has a clean, pleasant scent, and doesn't stain clothes.

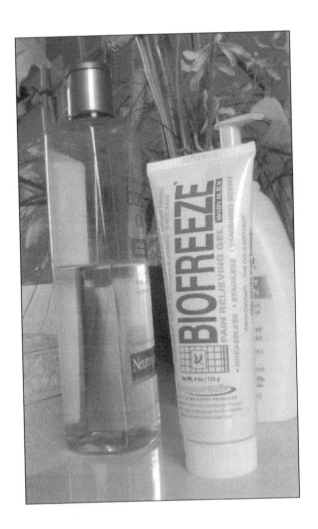

A Nine Step Program for Healing Your Arthritis

This 9-step program is based on the latest clinical research available. It gives you the best chance of healing your arthritis.

- Life is motion. Get your joints moving with chiropractic adjustments. Chiropractic care will also take abnormal stresses off your joints, helping them heal while preventing further degeneration.

- Clean up your diet. Healthy joints depend as much on good nutrition as any other part of your body. You will do better with a diet rich in fruits, vegetables, beans, whole grains, nuts, seeds and minimal junk food. So eat more fruits and vegetables. Cut out red meat as much as possible. Avoid sugar and tobacco, and minimize alcohol and caffeine. Also, drink 8 glasses of distilled water each day. Just cleaning up your diet will do wonders for your joints.

- Start taking a joint wellness formula containing glucosamine and other natural anti-inflammatory substances. Follow package directions.

- Start taking enzyme supplements. Follow package directions.

- Start taking Omega-3 supplements. Take 1500-3000mgs/day, depending on your weight (under/over 175lbs)

- Get on a stretching/exercise program. Water aerobics is the best exercise for most people, so find a pool with an aerobic program and jump in. No pool? Chapter Seven's "Dynamic Relaxer" is a great stretching program for arthritis sufferers. And use warmth. Warmth keeps the fluids moving in your joints. Hot tubs can be comforting, as can soaking in a warm bath for at least twenty minutes. Adding a cup each of Epsom salts and baking soda helps many people ease the joint pain of arthritis.

- Get enough rest. You might try taking a 10-20 minute nap after lunch if you aren't getting enough sleep at night.

- Start taking Vitamin C and Vitamin E—these are "building blocks" your body needs to keep joints healthy. Take 500mg of vitamin C three times/day; take 400 IU's of vitamin E each day. This step is especially important if you smoke, because smoking breaks down joint tissues. Vitamin C and E help protect against this breakdown.

- Start rubbing a pain-relieving topical ointment such as Biofreeze on your joints three times each day.

Help For Morning Energy

At one time there were Gypsies in places like Romania, Bulgaria and Transylvania. They didn't have villages of their own. They traveled in caravans from town to town, camping out in the deep, dark forests.

The Gypsies lived a good life, but they had a problem. There were bands of wild wolves that also roamed the forests. The wolves would prey on the gypsies. They'd come into camp and steal the food, bite the children and generally be a pain in the goulash. The gypsies had a terrible time fighting off these wolves.

Then one day the Gypsies built a big bonfire in the center of camp. They noticed that with this bonfire burning the wolves didn't attack. They said to themselves, "Hey, maybe we can start building bonfires instead of fighting wolves!" They did, and they got along much better.

Rather than waiting for health problems to attack, we need to concentrate on building the inner bonfire of health burning within each of us. If we do, we find the wolves of sickness and disease don't attack so much. The best time to start is now, by learning a simple morning wake-up routine.

Fire Starters

Many of us go through a morning ritual where we drag ourselves out of bed, then shock our nervous systems into alertness with coffee sweetened with sugar or with soft drinks. This sort of wake-up routine not only contributes to subluxations; it wears down our bodies faster than a milling stone grinding wheat.

Eating sugary foods in the morning for energy poses other problems. Many foods, including fruit and bread, contain basically the same chemical composition as candy. However, the sugar in a banana is gradually absorbed into your bloodstream. Sweets, on the other hand, rush into your blood, creating high levels of blood sugar, which if uncontrolled can lead to all kinds of nasty health problems.

To bring blood sugar levels down, your pancreas--a small gland tucked underneath your stomach--pours seven to ten times the normal amount of the chemical insulin into your bloodstream. Insulin takes the sugar from your blood and transfers it into your body's cells. Excess sugar is turned into shiny globs of fat, which is stored throughout your body.

Some experts think that after years of straining to keep you from turning your blood into a candy store the pancreas eventually "burns out". It loses the ability to produce adequate insulin, and you develop diabetes, a disease in which your body can't regulate blood sugar.

More Energy Without Caffeine or Sugar

You want to get off coffee, soft drinks and sugary sweets. But you need an energy boost! What can you do? Herbal teas are great alternatives. They can give you the clear-headedness and extra energy of a cup of coffee or a Coke, but without the ill-effects of caffeine and sugar.

Green tea is a powerful stimulant. Yes, it contains caffeine, but it also has health-giving antioxidants that have been shown to help fight cancer. In addition, it contains chemicals that lower cholesterol, and inhibit the formation of abnormal blood clots. Coffee has none of these positive effects, making green tea a better option when you need a pick me up.

Want to rid yourself of the caffeine habit completely? Ginseng and Gingko Biloba herbal teas are caffeine-free, brain-boosting, energy-lifting beverages. The best are the all-organic ones made by Yogi Teas. You'll be surprised at the coffee-like effects drinking these teas will have on you.

The Energy Roller Coaster

In Chapter Six we talked about how people who rely on coffee and sweets for energy put themselves on an energy roller coaster every day. In the morning they drink coffee or soda containing caffeine. This sends nerve impulses crackling through their bodies. (Remember those big sparks Dr. Frankenstein used to bring his monster to life?) In addition, the sugar in the coffee, soda or breakfast food dumps into the bloodstream, increasing blood sugar. Viola! Instant energy.

But within a few hours the caffeine wears off, blood sugar drops, and the person heads for the coffee pot, soda machine or snack bar.

Getting on such an energy roller coaster every day leads to mood and productivity swings and robs us of the chance to develop a natural inner abundance of energy. How do we build an "inner bonfire" of health and get off the energy roller coaster? Read on…

Wake Up, Tune In

How can you build an inner bonfire of health? One of the best ways is to enliven your nervous system with a morning wake-up routine. Think of this ritual as a tonic you can "take" every morning that will, over time, build a stronger nervous system.

The following routine is done in bed. Just prop a pillow comfortably behind your back and you're ready to start. Of course, you don't have to do it in bed. It works great as a warm-up before a regular morning exercise/stretching routine, or anytime you feel like refreshing yourself, in which case you can do the routine in a chair or cross-legged on the floor. As you move through the routine take deep, slow breaths. You'll start with your eyes and work down your body, ending at your feet.

The Eyes

- Rub your hands together for about 10 seconds until they begin to warm up. When you've generated some heat, use your hands to cup your eyes. Feel the warmth soak into your eyes for a few seconds.

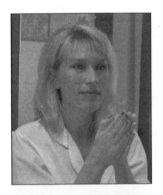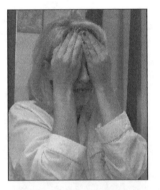

- Repeat three times.

- Now make fists with your hands and rub the sides of your index fingers together, again generating some heat. Use the inside part of the knuckles on your index fingers, and rub them over the tops of your eye sockets, starting near the bridge of the nose and moving outward. Make three quick strokes from the inside out. Rub the index fingers together again and make three strokes on the underside of your eye sockets.

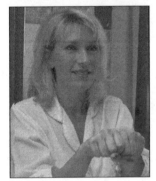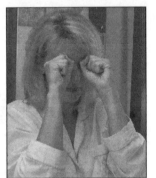

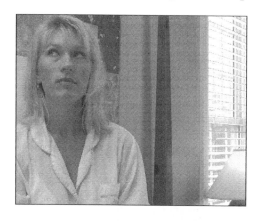

▪ Now it's time to stretch the muscles responsible for moving your eyes. Keeping your head straight and still, look up and to the right (see photo below). You should feel the muscles around your eyes stretch, just as if you were stretching a leg or arm. Keep looking up and to the right. Don't try to focus your eyes, just feel the stretch. Continue for about 10 seconds.

▪ Repeat looking up and to the left.

▪ Repeat looking down and to the left.

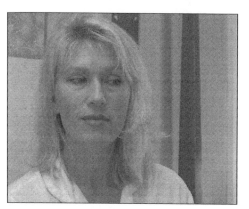

▪ Repeat again, looking down and right.

▪ Now, move your eyes in a circle. Start by looking straight up, then slowly move them clockwise to the right, down, left and up.

▪ Complete three circles.

▪ Repeat, moving your eyes counterclockwise.

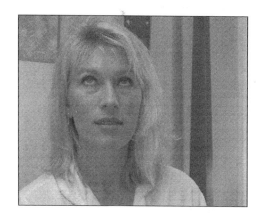

▪ Lastly, close your eyes, and using the tips of your fingers, gently massage your eyeballs with three slow, soft strokes, moving from the bridge of your nose to the corner of your eyes.

The Jaw, Tongue, Lips, Teeth, Mouth and Throat

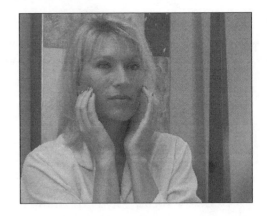

- Open your hands, spread your fingers, and using the tips of your fingers and thumb, tap your jaws, starting just below the ear and working down to the chin. Tap around the mouth and between the nose and lips, then move back up to just below the ears. Tap for 10-15 seconds.

- Next, with your mouth closed, move your tongue between your teeth and lips in a clockwise motion nine times. Now go counterclockwise nine times. Move the tongue inside the teeth and "wash" the inside of the teeth, nine times clockwise, nine counterclockwise. Note: your tongue may not be toned enough to make nine sweeps. If this is the case, start with four sweeps and build up to nine at your own pace.

- After all this tongue movement you will have built up a healthy supply of saliva in your mouth. Swallow this in three small sips.

- Lastly, gently click your teeth together 21 times. Do this fast, feeling the vibrations shake into your gums.

Note: The jaw/tongue movements outlined above loosen some of the most-used muscles and joints in the body. They are especially helpful to those suffering from TMJ (Temporomandibular Joint) problems, in which the jaw joints ache and click.

The Ears, Scalp and Cerebellum

- Now take your ears between your thumbs and forefingers and gently massage them, starting at the top and working down to the lobes. Take 10-15 seconds.

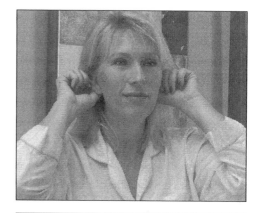

- Next, open your palms and spread your fingers, making your hands into "claws". Press your fingertips lightly into the hairline at your forehead and vigorously run your hands toward the back of your skull, running your fingers through your hair as you go. As you "brush" your hair, move your hands so that you cover the entire scalp. Make 48 strokes, increasing circulation to the scalp, improving your alertness.

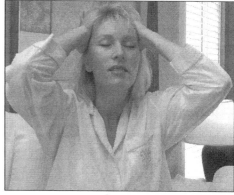

- Now cup your ears with the palms of your hands. Using your index and middle fingers, "flick" the middle finger against the back of your skull, using the index finger to first resist and then release the middle finger (the middle finger should "snap" off the index finger). This maneuver stimulates activity within the cerebellum, the part of your brain responsible for balance and coordination. It's an excellent tool to use whenever you need to quickly refocus your attention.

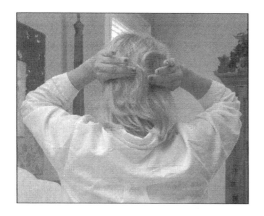

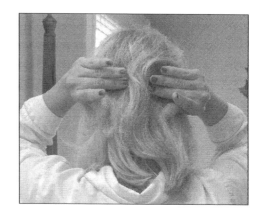

The Chest

- Making a fist with whichever hand feels more comfortable, lay your arm over your breastbone and raise and lower your fist in a thumping action against your chest. Bang the chest as hard as is comfortable. Repeat 21 times.

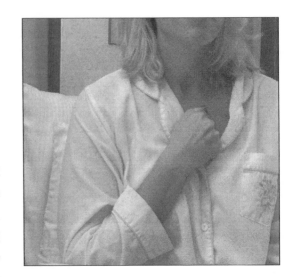

- Besides sending vibrations into the chest to stimulate airflow within the lungs, this maneuver stimulates the thymus gland. Tucked underneath our breastbone, this gland helps your body manufacture antibodies. By thumping your chest you'll stimulate your immune system.

Kidneys

- Sitting up straight, cup your hands, place them on your back about six to 10 inches up from your waist, and rub your back with an up and down motion.

- Rub for 10-15 seconds, heating the area. This gentle movement stimulates kidney function and is helpful in eliminating the waste products of digestion that have accumulated overnight.

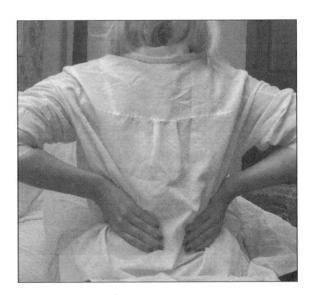

The Intestines and Colon

- Rub your hands together, generating heat. Cup whichever hand is most comfortable and place it on the skin just underneath your navel.

- Rub briskly in a clockwise motion 81 times, generating warmth. This movement awakens the "energy center" described in traditional Chinese medicine.

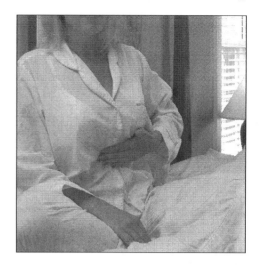

The Feet

- To complete the wake-up routine gently grasp your right foot with both hands and rub the foot in a wringing motion, starting with the heel/ankle and working your way up toward the toes. When the entire foot has been rubbed, push the toes forward, then bend them back. Repeat with the left foot.

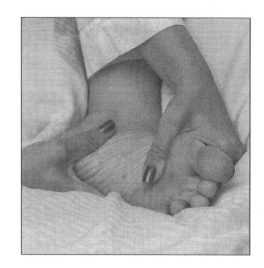

- If you have extra time, use your thumbs to gently massage the undersides of your feet, searching for any tender spots and spending 20 seconds or so massaging these tender areas. Massaging the feet not only prepares them for the rigors of pounding the pavement, but also stimulates the functions of many internal organs.

- To finish your wake-up routine close your eyes, take in a deep, slow breath...then slowly blow it out through your nose.

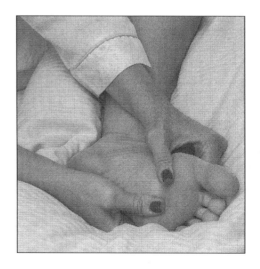

Help for Evening Peace

If you can't sleep it's difficult for your body to heal. Likewise, not sleeping depresses your immune system, predisposing you to illness.

So if sleep is so important, why do so many of us have a hard time getting the six to eight hours the typical person needs to thrive? There's no cookbook answer. What keeps you up may be entirely different than what keeps me staring at the ceiling. Pain keeps many awake, but the advice offered here is for those that don't hurt, they just can't sleep.

The best advice: Keep trying to find solutions that work for you. Try the tools and techniques listed here. Combine them if need be. Keep experimenting until you find an approach that works. The bottom line: even with a nighttime routine that usually gets you to sleep and keeps you sleeping, you'll still have nights when The Sandman just won't pay a visit. Many chronic insomniacs have found that praying or meditating at these times is the best way to spend their sleepless nights. Or you can make a list of activities you enjoy and engage in them when you can't sleep.

Here are the best strategies for getting to sleep and for sleeping through the night:

Exercise Hard Or Take A Walk After Dinner

Exercise is the best sleep tonic. Vigorous aerobic exercise in which you raise your heart rate to 70 percent of its maximum capacity induces deep sleep if done in the morning or afternoon hours. Exercising like that only a few hours before your bedtime, however, can keep you awake. So exercise hard and early in the day. If you can't, take a leisurely 20-minute walk after dinner. This practice will help you digest your food and produce muscle fatigue to help you sleep better.

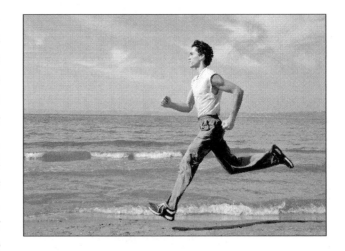

How To Create A Relaxing Bath

Soaking in a nice warm bath for 30 minutes to an hour before bed can be a great sleep tonic. When you get out of a warm tub your core body temperature, raised by being in the warm water, suddenly drops. This causes your heart rate and breathing to slow, creating a drowsy feeling. Here's how to turn your tub into a sleep-inducing tank.

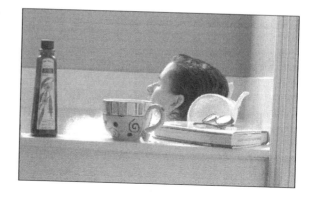

- Fill your tub with warm water. Don't make it hot, as hot water may be too stimulating.

- If your muscles are sore, add one cup of Epsom salt to the water. (Epsom salt contains large concentrations of magnesium, a natural muscle relaxer.)

- Add 5 drops of Lavender essential oil (available at natural food stores) to the water as the tub is filling. Lavender has been used for centuries as a natural tranquilizer by those practicing aromatherapy.

- Use scented candles to help create a tranquil setting. Candles containing the essential oil combination of lavender and ylang ylang are especially good for calming your senses.

- Add music to your "home spa". Inexpensive nature soundtracks featuring the sounds of the ocean, rainstorms or mountain streams can bring you back to a peaceful state.

Herbal Teas That Induce Sleep

Several herbal teas will help you fall asleep (you might try sipping them while soaking in your relaxing bath). Two well-known brands are "Sleepy Time" by Celestial Seasons and "Bedtime" by Yogi Tea. Both contain a blend of teas that act as natural tranquilizers.

Chamomile is a popular herbal tea with a very pleasant taste that many find perfect for sipping before hitting the pillow. You can increase the sedative effects of any herbal tea by adding to it a tablespoon of Valerian Root extract (again, available at health food stores). This has a sweet, pungent taste that some like and others find really awful. If you don't like the taste of the extract, you can take Valerian Root capsules instead (see below).

Supplements To Help You Fall Asleep and Stay Asleep

Several products/supplements have proven to be very helpful to patients with sleep problems. They are listed here from least expensive to the priciest. I'd try the most economical first, as there isn't a correlation between the cost of a sleep supplement and its ability to get you to sleep. Again, what works for you may not work for me.

- Quietude by Borion is an inexpensive homeopathic remedy with no side effects. You just pop two of the sugary-tasting pills under your tongue when you go to bed.

- Valerian Root capsules. These are in the same price range as Quietude, but they can cause bad-tasting burps and make some people groggy the next morning. Most Valerian Root sold comes with a warning not to drive while taking this herbal tranquilizer. It's also available as a liquid extract.

- Passion Flower capsules. Similar to Valerian in their effect; they may work better for some people. It's also available as a liquid extract.

- Melatonin. This natural hormone is used by the body to regulate sleep. It seems to provide excellent results for short-term usage, but the sleep-promoting effects tend to wear off with consistent use.

- 5-HTP. This is a more expensive supplement. It's used by the brain to make Serotonin, a natural tranquilizer. If the supplements and herbs listed above don't work, don't give up on natural sleep aids until you've tried 5-HTP. It should be taken right before bed with three to four ounces of fruit juice or a third of an apple, banana or other fruit. (Taking it with one of these natural sources of carbohydrate helps get 5-HTP into your brain.) Don't take 5-HTP if you take prescription anti-depressants.

9 TRAINING DAYS
[designing your personal health program]

Personal Check

The exercises and other techniques in this book will create more health in your life. Virtually every adult first comes to our office because they are in pain. But then we teach them that true health is not the absence of pain or other symptoms, but a body and mind functioning at the very highest level possible.

> *If you wanted to win an Olympic gold metal in run-*
> *ning, could you make the Olympic team by running for*
> *five minutes a week? Anytime we want our bodies to do*
> *something better we have to train them. If you want*
> *your nervous system to work better you have to train it,*
> *too.*

Chiropractors do wonders, but the people coming into our clinics often bring problems they've had for many years, problems that only recently began producing noticeable symptoms. Working to correct the underlying problems takes time and effort, but in the end you may meet someone you haven't seen in a long time: A HEALTHY YOU!

Race Course

Life's fast pace can keep us from calming down. "Time stress"—feeling we don't have enough time to take care of ourselves—is one of the biggest barriers to natural living and natural health.

Not only does time pressure create stress, it prevents people from allowing their bodies to heal naturally. It pushes them toward therapies offering quick fixes that cover up symptoms rather than letting their bodies heal from the inside out.

Often patients will come to my office in pain. Many—most, in fact—will take awhile to heal. Some will come in on their second or third visit and say something like, "My back is still hurting!" As if one or two visits could erase years of degenerative changes in their spine. Whether their pain began suddenly or developed over years, most patients want it gone NOW!

When patients present this attitude I ask them if they like to eat spaghetti. Most say yes. I'll ask how long it takes for spaghetti to cook. They say "about ten minutes".

"That's right," I'll say. "You know, I'd love for my spaghetti to cook in two minutes, but Mother Nature doesn't care what I think. She's going to take 10 minutes to cook my spaghetti. That's because every process in nature requires time. Nature has a timetable for everything. It's the same with your body. Once we get your nervous system functioning correctly we have to wait for Nature to do the healing. That may happen quickly or slowly, but we can't control it. Give Nature the time she needs."

"The impulse frequently arises in me to squeeze another this or another that into this moment. Just this phone call, just stopping off here on my way there. Never mind that it might be in the opposite direction. I've learned to identify this impulse and mistrust it. I work hard at saying no to it...I like to practice voluntary simplicity to counter such impulses... Voluntary simplicity means going fewer places in one day rather than more, seeing less so I can see more, doing less so I can do more, acquiring less so I can have more..."

From "Wherever You Go There You Are"
by Jon Kabat-Zinn

Training Table

You're about to develop a training program. You'll follow a three-step process. *First* you'll identify the exercises and techniques best suited to your current condition. *Next* you'll review your schedule and find time to use this book's ideas. *Finally* you'll write a schedule for **this week** so you can start training.

In developing a personal training program, first consider if you are currently in pain. What part or parts of your body hurt the worst?

Nightmare Neck

If you're dealing with neck pain and/or headaches your training should emphasize Chapter Four's neck pain relief routine. Here are some guidelines:

- ***DO NOT DO ANY EXERCISE THAT CAUSES YOU PAIN***. Typically you'll be able to do all the exercises if you're gentle with yourself. Do very small movements at first, increasing them until you reach a pain threshold, then back off. **AGAIN, AS SOON AS YOU FEEL PAIN DECREASE YOUR MOVEMENTS.**

- Pushing yourself into the pain zone when exercising is counterproductive. When your body sends pain signals to your brain, your brain responds by tightening muscles in that area of your body. So if your neck is hurting and you stretch and cause pain, the neck muscles may become tighter.

- Generally you should follow the number of repetitions given with each exercise. If you enjoy a particular exercise you can increase the number of repetitions as your neck pain begins to fade.

- If you find certain exercises relieve your pain symptoms better than others, by all means spend more time on them. Likewise, leave out any exercises that aggravate your condition.

- Breathing deeply and slowly is as important when doing the exercises as the exercises themselves. Let your breath help relax your muscles.

- If your neck or back pain is chronic in nature, use heat to relax the area and bring it more blood flow. For the neck, shoulders and back, apply heat for twenty minutes at a time. In the wrists, elbows, ankles and knees, fifteen minutes. If your pain is the result of an injury or over use (gardening for the first time during the Spring, or helping your friend load his moving truck), where you've strained your muscles, use ice for the same amount of time noted above for the first three days; then use heat.

If headaches are your main problem do the Trigger Fingers technique two times each day, in the morning upon awakening and at night, before bed. Do the technique before your neck exercises to make them more effective. You'll also want to try the techniques outlined in the "Special Help For Your Headaches" section.

Also helpful if you're suffering from headaches and/or neck pain are Chapter Seven's relaxation techniques. Practicing The Quiet Mind routine can often give you a different perspective on your pain, providing some distance from it, making it more manageable.

If your neck pain is not accompanied by headaches, concentrate on the stretching exercises and the self-massage technique. Perform self-massage on your neck and shoulders at least three times a day at work to help relieve the strain of sitting at a desk. Take a break from your chores every hour or two to stretch and massage. This need only take two or three minutes, and can coincide with bathroom breaks and mealtimes so you don't feel time pressure.

The warmth of a relaxing bath containing a de-stressing essential oil will help relax your neck muscles, and when used in conjunction with self massage can help break the spasm/pain/spasm cycle at the root of many neck pains (see "Help For Evening Peace" in the Special Help section). In addition, natural supplements for muscle and joint pain should also be a cornerstone of your program. And don't forget the advice in Chapter Six's "Eating To Get Out Of Pain" section. You'll want to start eating to feel better right away.

Back Bitten

If you're back hurts concentrate on Chapter Five's back pain relief program. All the advice given above for doing the neck pain relief exercises applies to your back as well. Be as gentle with your back as possible when doing the exercises, and de-stress as often as you can with relaxing baths and hot packs. (Note: you can buy re-useable hot/cold packs at a pharmacy. Microwave for one minute on "High," and wrap in a moist, thin dish towel. Apply to your back for 20 minutes every hour that your schedule allows. Again, if your back has been injured, use ice rather than heat for the first three days.) It's best to do your exercises after having used heat or ice.

If your job requires lifting, twisting or other motions that make your back hurt, talk to your supervisor about doing light duty work until your back is feeling better. The same advice goes for household chores. When possible, get help lifting small children.

Many people with back pain try to live with it, going about their normal daily routine, and end up severely injuring themselves. Most back operations occur after a person has had many warning signs from their back, but they've chosen to ignore them. One day the dam breaks. The person winds up under the knife because their back has degenerated beyond the point of rehabilitation. While low back pain may come and go, most low back *problems* don't improve with time, only with care.

Your back may recuperate faster if you wear a back brace while driving and doing other activities (see the "Back (Brace) Talk" section in Chapter Five).

Above And Beyond

In time you should reach a point where getting out of pain isn't your main concern. If you've had neck, headache or back problems for a long time you'll want to keep doing your favorite pain relief exercises every day. When you haven't experienced pain for four weeks you can pick one or two exercises and do them every other day. The 5 minutes you spend will condition your body against further relapses.

But you'll also want to practice other techniques to achieve higher health levels. As we've pointed out, just because you're out of pain doesn't mean you're healthy. To achieve higher levels of health you'll want to start using some of the other tools we've talked about. Here are some ideas:

- A good place to start building your inner bonfire of health is at the table. Nutrition so powerfully affects your health that you'll want to get this piece of the health puzzle into place as quickly as possible. Don't try to change all your eating habits overnight; incorporate as many of Chapter Six's suggestions as are comfortable.

- You'll also need to work on your breathing, so incorporate "Breath of Fire" and "Belly Breathing" exercises into your daily routine.

- It's also a great time to try a wake-up routine (see "Help For Morning Energy" in the Special Help section).

- If you're not participating in an aerobic activity such as running, walking, swimming or bicycling, now is an excellent time to start. Get your heart pumping for at least 25 minutes, three times each week. Any of these changes will impact your health like a freight train full of positive energy.

- If you work at a desk or notice that, over the years, your shoulders have rounded and your head has dropped forward, you'll find Chapter Four's Perfect Posture program especially helpful. With daily practice you should notice postural changes within a month or two. Even doing one or two of the exercises at your desk throughout the day will help prevent your neck and shoulders from becoming stiff and sore.

- Chapter Seven's Dynamic Relaxer is particularly rejuvenating. Do it as part of a morning wake-up ritual or as a warm-up before athletic or aerobic activities.

Optimally, in addition to your regular chiropractic adjustments, your personal program will include:

- A morning wake-up routine that includes stretching exercises.

- Eating for optimal nutrition and pain control, including supplementing your diet with herbs and vitamins.

- A regular aerobic conditioning program.

- Time out for relaxing and working on your mind/body connection.

Sound like a lot? Actually you can do all this in about an hour spread throughout your 14-hour day. The key is to make health a lifestyle. You may not be able to cram more activities into your present life. Instead, start replacing some of the things you're doing now with the activities described in this book. If you do, better health is sure to come to you.

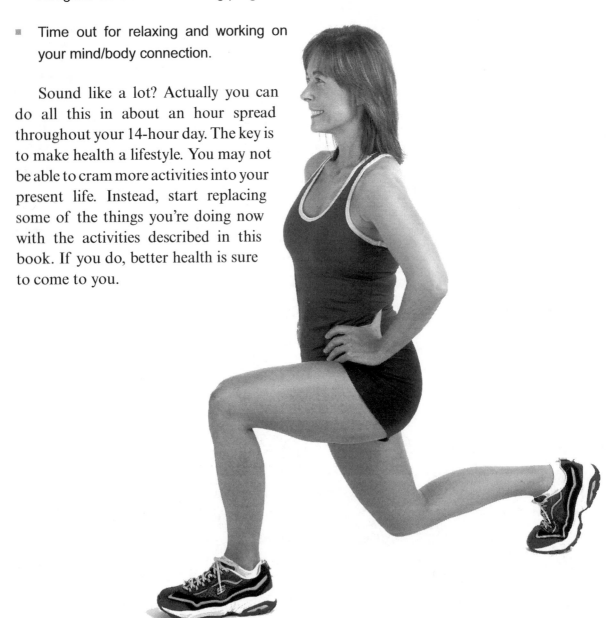

3 Steps to Better Health

[designing your personal health training program]

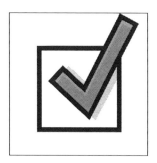

**Choose Your Exercise And
Other Self-Help Tools**

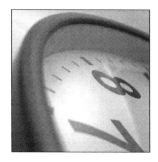

Identify Training Time

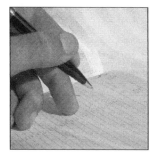

Plan Your Program

STEP 1:

Choose the exercises and other techniques for your personal program.

Chapter 4

Posing Problems

Neck Pain Relief

☐ Basic Neck Stretch
☐ Basic Neck Stretch Using A Chair
☐ The Shoulder Shrug
☐ Shoulder Shrug Two
☐ The Reader
☐ Trigger Fingers
☐ Trigger Fingers With A Partner
☐ Self Massage
☐ Resistance Stretching
☐ Using Tennis Balls For Tension Headaches/Upper Neck Pain
☐ Using Tennis Balls For Lower Neck Pain

The Perfect Posture Program

☐ The Ball Bearing
☐ The Back Loop
☐ The Wall Slide
☐ The Turtle
☐ Tips For Getting And Keeping Good Posture

Chapter 5

Pelvic Power

Back Pain Relief

☐ The Knee Pull Stretch
☐ The Deep Tilt
☐ The Side-To-Side

Ch 5 continued. . .

☐ The Bicycle
☐ The Back Builder
☐ Using Tennis Balls For Back Pain/Sciatica
☐ Stomach Crunches
☐ Sitting Back Stretch
☐ How To Lift
☐ Is A Back Brace Right For You?

Chapter 6

High Voltage

Energy Eating Etiquette

☐ Eat Food In Its Natural State
☐ Drink Enough Water
☐ Eat Less
☐ Eat In A Peaceful Atmosphere
☐ Eat In A Comfortable Position
☐ Eat Only When You Are Hungry
☐ Avoid Ice Cold Or Piping Hot Food And Drink
☐ Chew Food Slowly And Thoroughly
☐ Limit How Much You Drink With Your Food
☐ Bless Your Food

Killing You Harshly

☐ Sugar and Sugar Substitutes
☐ Artificial Food Additives And Preservatives
☐ Junk Food
☐ Too Many Dairy Products
☐ Too Much Meat
☐ Too Much Caffeine

174

Ch 6 continued. . . .

Handling Digestion Problems
- [ ] Proper Food Combining
- [ ] Using Enzymes
- [ ] Using Probiotics
- [ ] Fixing "Leaky Gut Syndrome"
- [ ] Eating Enough Fiber
- [ ] Detoxification Programs

Vitamins for Nervous System Health
- [ ] Multivitamin/Mineral Supplements

Nerve Herbs
- [ ] Ginkgo Biloba
- [ ] Ginseng

Blockbuster Supplements for Specific Health Issues
- [ ] Adrenal Gland Support
- [ ] Joint Support
- [ ] Help For Sore Muscles
- [ ] Natural Anti-Inflammatories
- [ ] Brain Food
- [ ] Growth Hormone Releasing
- [ ] Supplements
- [ ] Cholesterol Lowering Supplements
- [ ] Protein Drinks

Ch 6 continued. . .

Eating to Get out of Pain
- [ ] Creating A Basic pH Environment
- [ ] Avoiding Processed Foods

Eating and Breathing for Energy
- [ ] Diet And The Hyperactive Child
- [ ] Using Protein To Think More Clearly
- [ ] Breath Of Fire

Eating and Breathing to Relax
- [ ] Eating Carbohydrates To Relax
- [ ] Slow Belly Breathing

Chapter 7
Block Busters

Mind/Body Health
- [ ] Training To Stay Young
- [ ] The Dynamic Relaxer
- [ ] The Quiet Mind Technique
- [ ] Communicating With Your Symptoms
- [ ] The Trauma Release Process

Chapter 8
Special Help

Help For Your Feet
- ☐ Using A Tennis Ball
- ☐ Using A Frozen Water Bottle
- ☐ Stretching Your Arches With A Towel
- ☐ Scrunching Up A Towel
- ☐ Soaking/Pampering Your Feet

Help For Your Knees
- ☐ Straight Leg Raise With A Towel
- ☐ Straight Leg Raise
- ☐ Leg Lunges
- ☐ Toe Raises
- ☐ The Calf Stretch
- ☐ The Quadriceps Stretch
- ☐ The Hamstring Stretch

Help For Your Hips
- ☐ Squatting Hip Stretch
- ☐ Basic Hip Stretch
- ☐ Basic Hip Stretch Two
- ☐ Hip Stretch On A Bed
- ☐ Hip Stretch With A Belt
- ☐ Using Tennis Balls For Hip Pain

Help for Your Elbows and Wrists
- ☐ Basic Elbow/Wrist Stretch
- ☐ Wrist Curls
- ☐ Wrist Lifts
- ☐ Self Massage For Your Elbows

Help For Your Shoulders
- ☐ Shoulder Stretch One
- ☐ Shoulder Stretch Two
- ☐ The Pendulum Swing
- ☐ Wall Walking
- ☐ Rubber Tubing Exercises
- ☐ Corner Push Ups
- ☐ Using Tennis Balls For Shoulder Pain
- ☐ Threading The Needle

Help For Your Headaches
- ☐ Dietary Factors
- ☐ Relaxation And Exercise
- ☐ Trigger Point Work
- ☐ Using Ice Water
- ☐ Using Pressure
- ☐ Using Peppermint
- ☐ Using Magnesium

Help For Your Sinuses
- ☐ The Magic Of The Neti Pot
- ☐ Breathing Easier With Acupressure

Help for your Arthritis
- ☐ Glucosamine Sulfate
- ☐ Omega-3 Fatty Acids
- ☐ Enzyme Supplements
- ☐ Pain Relief Ointments
- ☐ A Nine-Step Program For Healing Your Arthritis

Help for Morning Energy
- ☐ Wake Up, Tune In
- ☐ The Jaw, Tongue, Lips, Teeth, Mouth And Throat
- ☐ The Ears, Scalp And Cerebellum
- ☐ The Chest
- ☐ Kidneys
- ☐ The Intestines And Colon
- ☐ The Feet

Help For Evening Peace
- ☐ Exercise To Sleep Better
- ☐ How To Create A Relaxing Bath
- ☐ Herbal Teas That Induce Sleep
- ☐ Supplements That Help You Fall Asleep And Stay Asleep

STEP 2:

> *Identify available training time.*

Morning	
☐ Before breakfast	*Notes:*
☐ In the shower	
☐ During morning commute to work	
☐ Bathroom breaks	
☐ Work breaks	

Afternoon	
☐ Lunch	*Notes:*
☐ Bathroom breaks	
☐ Work breaks	

Evening	
☐ During evening commute from work	*Notes:*
☐ Before dinner	
☐ At the dinner table	
☐ During an evening bath	
☐ While reading, watching television	
☐ In the shower	
☐ In bed, before going to sleep	

STEP 3:

Make your training schedule.

MONDAY

MORNING	
AFTERNOON	
EVENING	

TUESDAY

MORNING	
AFTERNOON	
EVENING	

WEDNESDAY

MORNING	
AFTERNOON	
EVENING	